Mood and Anxiety Disorders in Children and Adolescents

A psychopharmacological approach

Mood and Anxiety Disorders in Children and Adolescents

A psychopharmacological approach

David Nutt
Caroline Bell
Christine Masterson
Clare Short

Martin Dunitz

© 2001 Martin Dunitz Ltd, a member of the Taylor & Francis group

First published in the United Kingdom in 2001 by
Martin Dunitz Ltd
The Livery House
7-9 Pratt Street
London NW1 0AE

Tel: +44-(0)20-7482-2202
Fax: +44-(0)20-7267-0159
E-mail: info.dunitz@tandf.co.uk
Website: http://www.dunitz.co.uk

A CIP catalogue record for this book is available from the British Library

ISBN 1-85317-924-8

Distributed in the USA by
Fulfilment Center
Taylor & Francis
7625 Empire Drive
Florence, KY 41042, USA
Toll Free Tel: 1-800-634-7064
E-mail: cserve@routledge_ny.com

Distributed in Canada by
Tayor & Francis
74 Rolark Drive
Scarborough
Ontario M1R 4G2, Canada
Toll Free Tel: 1-877-226-2237
E-mail: tal_fran@istar.ca

Distributed in the rest of the world by
ITPS Limited
Cheriton House
North Way, Andover
Hampshire SP10 5BE, UK
Tel: +44 (0) 1264 332424
E-mail: reception@itps.co.uk

Composition by Wearset, Boldon, Tyne and Wear
Printed and bound in Great Britain by Biddles Ltd, Guildford and King's Lynn

Contents

About the authors

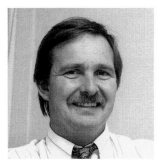

David Nutt

David Nutt is currently Professor of Psychopharmacology and Dean of Clinical Medicine and Dentistry, in the University of Bristol. He is also a member of the Advisory Council on the Misuse of Drugs, the MRC Neuroscience Advisory Board and the CSM (Committee on Safety of Medicines). In addition, he is Advisor to the British National Formulary, the editor of the *Journal of Psychopharmacology* and the Past-President of the British Association of Psychopharmacology. His particular research interests include the areas of anxiety, depression, sleep and addiction.

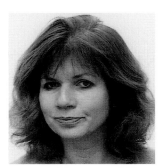

Caroline Bell

Caroline Bell is a Specialist Registrar in General Adult Psychiatry and a research fellow at the Psychopharmacology Unit, Bristol University. Her research interest has been in the field of the psychopharmacology of anxiety and depression. This has involved work on projects examining the role of serotonin in these disorders and clinical studies testing the efficacy of drugs in the treatment of these conditions in adults.

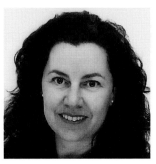

Christine Masterson

Christine Masterson is a Consultant Child and Adolescent Psychiatrist based within a multidisciplinary team at Ashford and St Peter's NHS Trust, Chertsey, Surrey. Her interests include paediatric liaison and psychopharmacology.

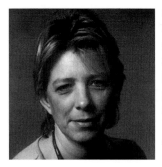

Clare Short

Clare Short is a Specialist Registrar on the Child and Adolescent Psychiatry training scheme in Bristol. During her training she has balanced the clinical practice of these disciplines by developing knowledge and experience in both the biological aspects of mental illness together with the practice of psychotherapeutic techniques.

1
Introduction

This book discusses the current state of knowledge of mood and anxiety disorders in children and adolescents from a psychopharmacological perspective and gives clinicians practical advice on the use of medication in this age group. This is a rapidly evolving field, and it is apparent that many questions remain unanswered. What is clear, however, is that a psychopharmacological way of thinking often provides a useful model for explaining the nature of disorders to children and their families, why they need to take medication, and how these drugs may work. For the clinician, a similar understanding makes the process of knowing why, when, what, and how to prescribe much more logical.

Recent advances have led to a rapid increase in our knowledge of the neurobiological processes underlying these conditions. This has been paralleled by an ever-increasing number of available treatment options appearing on the market. Choosing the right drug or therapy for each child may at first seem a daunting prospect, but understanding the psychopharmacology and neurochemistry involved makes the choice much more straightforward. Of course, there is nothing quite like clinical experience; but this in combination with a scientific approach means that treatment can be tailored to specific symptoms and disease profiles, and side-effects can be anticipated and explained.

Although in this book we concentrate on psychopharmacological approaches, we are not advocating the use of drug treatments in isolation or their use in every young person. Medication is most effective when incorporated into a carefully thought-out management plan based on a clearly established diagnosis. The key to this is a thorough assessment of all the factors involved (psychological, biological and social) and the impact these have on every area of the child's life. This also includes time spent educating the child and family about the nature of the illness, the aetiological factors involved, the likely time course of recovery, and any potential side-effects that may be experienced. At least initially, youngsters should be seen frequently (i.e. once or twice weekly) during treatment to allow the careful monitoring of response and side-effects, and for titration of the drug up to a therapeutic level. Symptoms should be monitored throughout treatment in a standardized way, with, for example, self-rating scales to measure levels of severity and avoidance. These approaches have in common the theme of increasing patient understanding and compliance; and there is growing evidence that this type of approach adds to drug effects and facilitates recovery.

The first two chapters of this book give an overview of the important neurotransmitters involved in mood and anxiety disorders and the mechanisms of action and side-effect profiles of the various drugs available for treatment. The following chapters describe the key features of each disorder, emphasizing the important factors which help the diagnostic process. For each disorder, important aetiological factors will be highlighted and linked to the psychopharmacological treatment options. We will then give a practical description of the use of medication in the different conditions, including the choice of drug, dose and duration of treatment, and what to do if patients fail to respond.

2
The basics

This chapter explains some of the basic concepts that are important to allow an understanding of many of the biological abnormalities found in the psychiatric disorders and how the drugs used to treat them work.

Neurones and how they function

In the central nervous system (CNS), information is transferred along neurones in the form of electrical impulses or action potentials which pass from the cell body to the terminal region of the nerve. It is here transformed into chemical information in the form of neurotransmitters (called first messengers). Following the arrival of an action potential, the vesicles where the neurotransmitter is stored undergo exocytosis, resulting in release of neurotransmitter into the synapse, where it is available to interact with postsynaptic receptors. The neurotransmitter is then either metabolized or taken back into the cell by reuptake processes *(Figure 1)*.

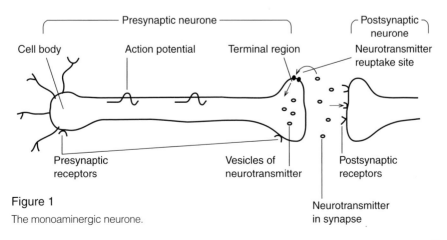

Figure 1

The monoaminergic neurone.

The interaction of the neurotransmitter with postsynaptic receptors accounts for the therapeutic and adverse effects of most psychotropic drugs. These postsynaptic receptors are linked to either (1) ion channels or (2) protein complexes called G-proteins (so named because of their ability to bind the guanine nucleotides, guanosine triphosphate (GTP) or diphosphate (GDP)). Receptors which are linked to ion channels produce rapid responses, while those linked to the G-proteins trigger a cascade of reactions and therefore slower responses *(Figure 2)*. Activation of G-proteins leads to production of second messengers (e.g. cyclic adenosine monophosphate (cAMP), cyclic guanosine monophosphate (cGMP), phosphatidylinositol), each of which has a specific affinity for a member of another group of intracellular proteins called protein kinases. When activated these kinases phosphorylate specific proteins to produce third messengers which then produce a wide variety of effects including changing cell metabolism, cell division and gene expression.

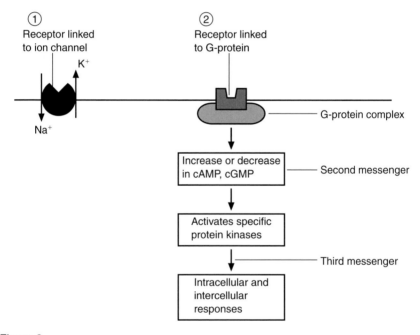

Figure 2

Postsynaptic receptor effects.

The neurotransmitters

Our present knowledge suggests that in mood and anxiety disorders the important neurotransmitters are noradrenaline (NA), serotonin (5-HT), dopamine (DA) and γ-aminobutyric acid (GABA). This section summarizes how each neurotransmitter is synthesized and metabolized, their principal receptors and major pathways in the brain.

Noradrenaline

NA is synthesized from the amino acid tyrosine which is actively pumped into the NA neurone *(Figure 3)*. It is first transformed into DOPA by the enzyme tyrosine hydroxylase (the rate-limiting and most important step in the regulation of NA synthesis), then into DA by DOPA decarboxylase and finally into NA by dopamine β-hydroxylase. It is then stored in vesicles until released into the synapse by the arrival of an action potential. NA is then removed from the synapse by a specific pump for NA (the NA reuptake pump or transporter) which transports NA into the cell where it is available to be stored again or metabolized. The metabolism of NA is by two enzymes, monoamine oxidase (MAO) and catechol-*O*-methyl-transferase (COMT), which produce the end products 3-methoxy-4-hydroxyphenylglycol (MHPG) and vanillymandelic acid (VMA).

There are three important receptors for NA in the CNS – α_1, α_2 and β_1. All three are located on the postsynaptic neurone *(Figure 4)*. Some specific functions have been described for these which explain some of the side-

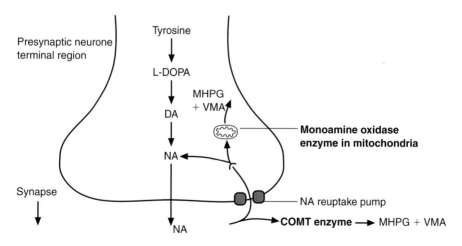

Figure 3

Synthesis and metabolism of NA.

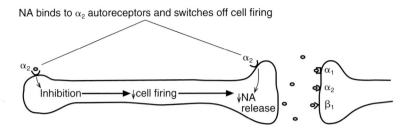

Figure 4
NA receptors.

effects of drugs, e.g. blockade of α_1 receptors producing postural hypotension (discussed further in Chapter 3). The α_2 receptors are predominantly peripheral being located in blood vessels, the pulmonary tree and GI tract.

The α_2 receptor, in addition to being present on the postsynaptic neurone, is also located on the presynaptic cell body and terminal region. Here it is called an autoreceptor, because it has the effect of regulating NA release through a negative feedback loop *(Figure 4)*. NA at this receptor produces inhibition of cell firing, so that when increased NA is present there is an increased inhibition of firing, which results in a subsequent reduction in NA release.

NA is widely projected in the CNS, which explains its involvement in a variety of functions *(Figure 5)*. The major site of the NA cell bodies is in

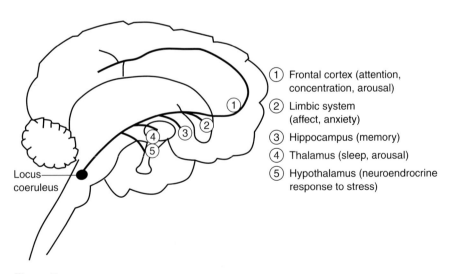

Figure 5
Major NA pathways in the brain.

the locus coerulus in the midbrain. Projections arise from here and are distributed to: (1) the frontal cortex (where they are presumed to have a role in attention, concentration and arousal) and from where they spread to other parts of the cortex; (2) the limbic system (involvement in affect and anxiety); (3) the hippocampus (involvement in memory and affect); (4) the hypothalamus (role in coordination of the neuroendocrine response to stress); and (5) the thalamus (involvement in arousal and sleep).

Serotonin

Serotonin is synthesized from the amino acid tryptophan, which is actively transported into the 5-HT neurone *(Figure 6)*. It is converted into 5-hydroxytryptophan (5-HTP) by the enzyme tryptophan hydroxylase (the rate-limiting step) and then into 5-HT by the enzyme aromatic acid decarboxylase. It is then stored in vesicles in the terminal region of the cell until released by the arrival of an action potential. As with NA and DA, there is a specific 5-HT transporter in the cell membrane which actively pumps 5-HT from the synapse into the neurone where it is destroyed by the MAO enzyme and converted into 5-hydroxyindoleacetic acid (5-HIAA).

At least seven subclasses of 5-HT receptor have so far been identified, many with several subtypes that subserve different and specific functions. At the moment three subclasses appear to be particularly important in psychiatry – the 5-HT_1, 5-HT_2 and 5-HT_3 receptors, with all three being found on the postsynaptic neurone *(Figure 7)*. Some specific functions

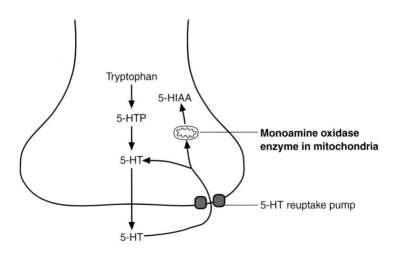

Figure 6
Synthesis and metabolism of 5-HT.

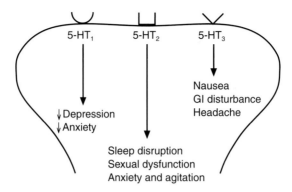

Figure 7
5-HT postsynaptic receptors.

have been determined for these receptors. Stimulation of 5-HT$_1$ receptors seems to be important in bringing about response in the treatment of depression and anxiety. Stimulation of 5-HT$_2$ receptors produces sleep disruption, sexual dysfunction and an increase in anxiety/agitation. Stimulation of 5-HT$_3$ receptors produces nausea, diarrhoea and headache. These effects explain many of the beneficial and adverse effects seen with drugs that increase 5-HT, e.g. SSRIs, which are discussed in Chapter 3.

In addition to their location on postsynaptic neurones, 5-HT$_1$ receptors are also found presynaptically. Here there are two subtypes – the 5-HT$_{1A}$ receptor, which is found on the cell body, and the 5-HT$_{1B/D}$ receptor, which is located on the terminal region of the neurone. At these sites they both function as autoreceptors which, like the α_2 receptor in the NA system, produce inhibitory effects when stimulated by the neurotransmitter. They thus form part of a negative feedback loop; increases in 5-HT results in an increased binding to these receptors which has an inhibitory effect thereby reducing cell firing and the release of 5-HT into the synapse *(Figure 8)*.

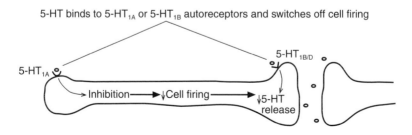

Figure 8
5-HT$_{1A}$ and 5-HT$_{1B}$ autoreceptors.

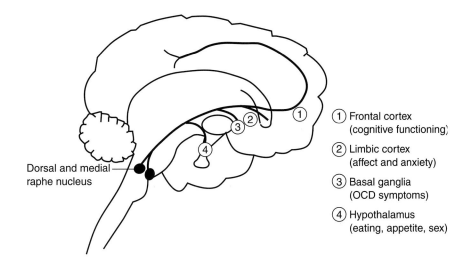

Figure 9
Major 5-HT pathways in the brain.

Like NA, 5-HT is also distributed widely in the brain. Projections go from the two raphe nuclei in the midbrain to (1) the prefrontal cortex (involvement in cognitive functioning) and from here to other parts of the cortex; (2) the limbic cortex (involvement in affect and anxiety); (3) the basal ganglia (explains some of the symptoms of obsessive compulsive disorder (OCD)); and (4) the hypothalamus (involvement in eating, appetite and sexual functioning) *(Figure 9)*.

Dopamine

DA is produced in DA neurones by the same pathway as NA and is destroyed by the same enzymes *(Figure 3)*. As with the other monoamines, there is also a specific DA transporter which actively pumps DA back into the presynaptic cell.

At least five DA receptors have been found so far, all of which are located postsynaptically *(Figure 10)*. Again, specific functions have been described for some of these. Perhaps the most important of these is the D_2 receptor, blockade of which is found to be beneficial in the treatment of psychosis.

There are three major sites of DA cell bodies in the CNS *(Figure 11)*. These are the substantia nigra, the ventral tegmental area (VTA) of the midbrain and the hypothalamus. Four major pathways project from these

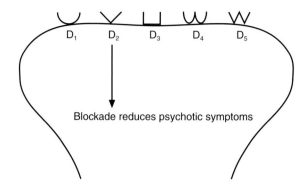

Figure 10
DA receptors.

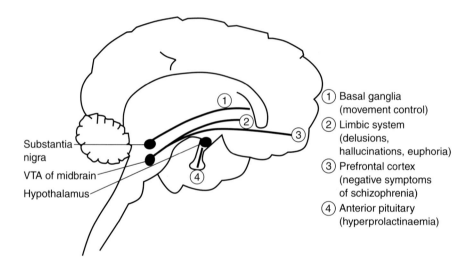

Figure 11
Major DA pathways in the brain.

sites and explain a variety of DA effects. These are: (1) the mesocortical pathway from the VTA to the prefrontal cortex, which explains the involvement of DA in the negative symptoms of schizophrenia. It also explains some of the cognitive side-effects produced by antipsychotics; (2) the mesolimbic pathway from the VTA to the nucleus accumbens in the limbic system, which explains its role in the production of delusions, hallucinations and the euphoric effects of drugs of abuse; (3) the nigrostriatal pathway from the substantia nigra to the basal ganglia, which explains the involvement of DA in the control of movement and extrapyramidal effects; and (4) the tuberoinfundibular pathway from the hypothalamus to the anterior pituitary, which inhibits prolactin release and explains the hyperprolactinaemia and related effects (e.g. gynaecomastia) of D_2 receptor-blocking antipsychotics.

GABA

GABA is the main inhibitory neurotransmitter in the brain. There are two types of GABA receptor – GABA-A and GABA-B. The GABA-A receptor is a postsynaptic macromolecular complex which spans the membrane. It forms a doughnut-like structure, with the hole in the centre being a pore through which chloride ions can pass *(Figure 12)*.

When GABA binds to this receptor it opens the central pore; this allows chloride ions to flow into the cell, hyperpolarizing the membrane and resulting in inhibition. As well as containing recognition sites for GABA, the complex also has specific sites for benzodiazepines, barbiturates and neurosteroids (derivatives of progesterone and cortisol).

GABA neurones are very widely distributed in the brain, with GABA-A receptors being found in the limbic system (amygdala, hippocampus), cerebellum, striatum and cortex.

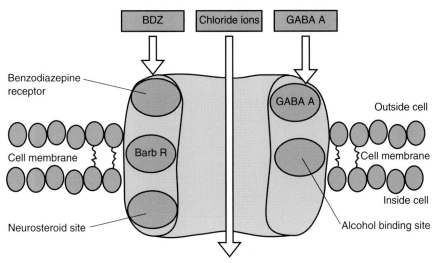

Barb = Barbiturate
R = Receptor

Figure 12
GABA-A receptor complex.

Interactions between neurotransmitters

Interactions exist at the neuronal level between all these four neurotransmitters. This means that changes in one neurotransmitter can lead to changes in the availability of another. This will be discussed further in Chapter 3.

Neurotransmitters and development

Major morphological changes clearly occur in the brain during development. Current thinking suggests that for some reason more neurons are produced than necessary, and that these must then be destroyed to reach the optimum level. Failure to achieve this has been associated with psychotic disorders, e.g. schizophrenia, when an excess of neurons has been reported in the frontal lobes. There is, however, no good evidence for a similar involvement in affective disorders.

Relatively little work has been done on the development of the neurotransmitter systems, although recent techniques involving the use of genetically modified animals have shed some light on the issue. For example, mice which have been genetically modified to lack 5-HT transporter proteins (5-HT transporter knockout mice) have been found to have increased 5-HT in the synapse. They have also been reported to be anxious and to have abnormal development of the sensory cortex relating to the whiskers (whisker cortex).

Another model which uses mice without 5-HT_{1A} receptors (5-HT_{1A} receptor knockout mice) has shown that this also has the effect of increasing 5-HT in the synapse and producing anxious mice. Of great interest to developmental theories is the recent observation that if the 5-HT abnormality is rectified in juvenile mice they become normal. If, however, they are not treated until adulthood the mice remain permanently anxious.

This suggests that 5-HT in childhood may play an important role in the development and regulation of adult psychopathology. This also fits with the considerable evidence of the impact of early trauma on the development of adult mood disorders.

Much less is known about the other neurotransmitter systems (NA, DA, acetylcloline) although it may well be that similar mechanisms are important.

3
Drugs and how they work

More and more drugs are developed each year aimed at treating specific conditions and symptoms. They are becoming increasingly sophisticated in terms of their effects on particular receptor systems and as a result have generally more specific effects and are safer drugs than their older equivalents. They are being used increasingly in children and adolescents despite the fact that many drugs have not been specifically investigated in this age group which requires the clinician to prescribe off-licence. This can have the effect of making the doctor feel uncertain, although the actual purpose of a licence is to limit the claims that a pharmaceutical company can make rather than limit the clinician's ability to prescribe. It also means that the art of prescribing in this age group relies on the extrapolation of data from adult studies.

The lack of study and research of drugs in this age group results from a combination of two factors. The first dates from a split that certainly did exist in psychiatry, with clinicians adopting a particular approach either pharmacological or psychotherapeutic. The second is due to the fact that pharmaceutical companies generally carry out controlled trials in adult populations. This is often because of the greater prevalence of the conditions in this age group, and because of the issue of consent in children and adolescents. As a consequence, most drugs obtain a licence that excludes or contraindicates their use in children. The situation will only be improved by studies targetted specifically at the use of drugs in children and adolescents. This is an important aim for the future, and now a Food and Drug Administration (FDA) requirement for new drugs. In this endeavour the FDA has given companies the incentive that they can have exclusive licensing rights for an additional 6 months if they include paediatric studies in their dossier.

This chapter will discuss the important pharmacokinetic interactions that are known and that need to be considered when prescribing for children and adolescents. It will then describe salient pharmacodynamic effects.

- Pharmacokinetics: what the body does to the drug.
- Pharmacodynamics: what the drug does to the body (mostly the brain).

Pharmacokinetics

Understanding the pharmacokinetics and the differences which occur in children and adolescents helps to explain the possible problem areas and how potential drug–drug interactions can take place.

Absorption

Orally administered drugs can undergo a number of interactions during their passage through the gastrointestinal tract. The important factors that affect absorption are similar in adults and children over 1 year. They include: the gastrointestinal pH, which alters the lipid solubility of drugs and their subsequent diffusion across mucus membranes; the formation of large drug complexes which are then poorly absorbed; and factors that alter gut motility and as a result either enhance or delay gastric emptying.

Distribution

Once absorbed, drugs enter the liver via the portal circulation. They are metabolized to various extents (the first-pass effect), and are then distributed to the tissues via the systemic circulation. Two important factors can affect distribution: protein binding and the apparent volume of distribution (V_D).

Protein-binding properties reach adult values by the age of 1 year. Most drugs are bound to albumin and it is only the unbound fraction that is pharmacologically active. Significant drug–drug interactions are associated with drugs that are more than 90 per cent bound to plasma proteins because they can displace other drugs that are similarly bound.

Drugs are soluble in water or fat according to their physicochemical characteristics. A large V_D means that a drug is heavily taken up into fatty tissues. Although there are differences between the V_D in children and adults these differences are offset by concomitant changes in elimination.

Metabolism and the P_{450} system

Most psychotropic drugs are metabolized by the cytochrome P_{450} (CYP450) enzyme system in the liver. A large number of CYP450 enzymes exist, with three being particularly important for psychotropic medication – CYP1A2, CYP2D6 and CYP3A4. Not all individuals have all these enzymes; for example, up to 5 per cent of caucasians lack fully functional forms of the 2D6 enzyme. This makes them slow metabolizers of drugs that use this pathway which means that potentially high drug levels may be produced. The P_{450} enzymes can be inhibited or induced by certain drugs, which explains their importance in understanding potential drug interactions, some of which are shown in *Table 1*.

An example of a clinically relevant interaction is that produced by the combination of selective serotonin reuptake inhibitors (SSRIs) with tricyclic antidepressants (TCAs). The SSRIs (paroxetine, fluoxetine and, to a lesser extent, sertraline) are potent inhibitors of CYP2D6, and as a result inhibit the metabolism of TCAs. This means that high and potentially toxic TCA levels can be produced when the two types of drug are used together. It is important to remember that this effect can occur when one drug is being replaced by another and is dependent on factors such as the half-lives of the drugs and the presence of active metabolites.

Some drugs induce the P_{450} enzymes, i.e. increase their activity. This has the effect of increasing metabolism and resulting in lower drug levels. Carbamazepine is an important example of a drug that can do this. Interestingly, carbamazepine is metabolized by the same enzymes that it induces, which means that, over time, the dose may need to be increased to maintain plasma drug levels.

Excretion

Renal excretion is composed of three major steps – glomerular filtration, active tubular secretion and tubular reabsorption. These approximate to adult levels by the age of 6–12 months but can all be sites for potential drug interactions, e.g. concomitant use of nonsteroidal anti-inflammatory drugs.

Practical matters

Clinically liquid preparations are frequently used in paediatrics and consideration regarding the choice of drug, e.g. SSRI, needs to take this fact into account (*Table 5*). Supervision to ensure compliance and minimize misuse is important.

Table 1   Some effects on the P_{450} system.

	1A2 Enzyme	2D6 Enzyme	3A4 Enzyme
Inhibited by	Fluvoxamine Grapefruit juice	Paroxetine Fluoxetine Sertraline	Nefazodone Fluvoxamine
Drugs that use this for metabolism	Theophylline Clozapine	TCAs β-Blockers	Terfenadine

Pharmacodynamic effects of drugs

Antidepressants

Antidepressants are not only effective in the treatment of depression but are also used in a variety of other conditions, including panic disorder, OCD, social phobia, anorexia and bulimia nervosa.

Since the development of iproniazid in the 1950s, a new antidepressant group has been released almost every decade, with the result that there are now a huge number for the clinician to choose from *(Figure 13)*. It is important to understand the mechanisms of action of the individual drugs, their potential benefits, and their likely side-effects. From this, the clinician can tailor the treatment to the child and explain or avoid the precipitation of side-effects. Increasingly clinicians are avoiding the use of the older tricyclic drugs in this age group due to concerns about neuro and cardio toxicity. Alongside this, the development of the SSRIs makes their use almost obsolete.

Nonetheless, for each antidepressant group, we describe the mechanism of action, its effects on NA/5-HT availability in the synapse, the consequent effects on postsynaptic receptors, and the effects on other neurotransmitter systems that may cause additional side effects.

Tricyclic antidepressants

TCAs block the reuptake of 5-HT and NA into the presynaptic nerve terminal at the uptake sites shown in *Figure 14*. This increases the available concentration of these neurotransmitters at the synapse and around the cell body. This effect occurs within 24 h, although therapeutic benefits are usually not seen for 10–20 days. This delay may be explained by the time it takes for changes in receptor function to occur. For example, in the case of 5-HT, antidepressants block the reuptake transporters which are found on both the terminal regions of the neurone and the cell body *(Figure 15)*. This results in increased availability of 5-HT at both these sites. However, the effect of increased 5-HT around the cell body is that more binds to 5-HT_{1A} autoreceptors, which switch off cell firing and subsequent 5-HT release (Chapter 1). Over 2–3 weeks this autoreceptor desensitizes, which means that the inhibitory effect on cell firing is turned off. This then results in the desired effect, i.e. increased availability of neurotransmitter in the synapse. Similar changes in α_2 receptors occur with NA-uptake blockers.

All the TCAs block the reuptake of both 5-HT and NA but to varying degrees *(Figure 16)*. This explains their different efficacy in different conditions and some of their different side-effects. The more serotonergic TCAs (clomipramine, imipramine) are more effective in the treatment of disorders thought to have an underlying 5-HT abnormality (such as OCD

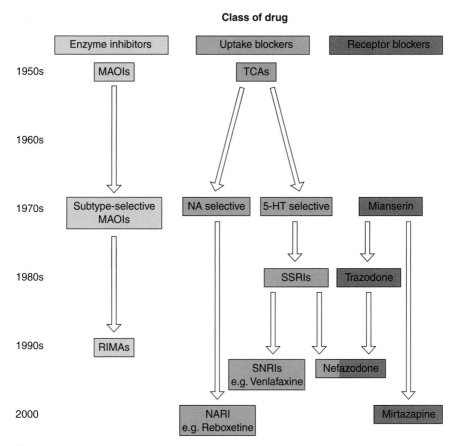

Figure 13

Available antidepressants.

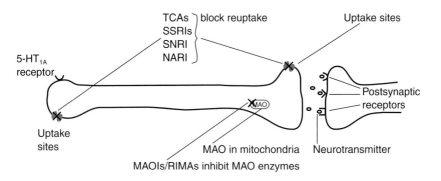

Figure 14

Sites of action of antidepressants.

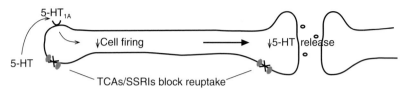

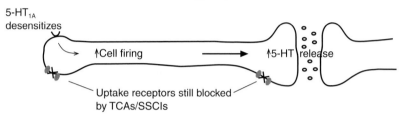

Figure 15

The 5-HT$_{1A}$ story.

or panic disorder). They are also associated with serotonergic side-effects, i.e. nausea, headache (5-HT$_3$ effects), and sexual dysfunction (5-HT$_2$ effects).

The adverse effects of TCAs are well known and can be understood in terms of their effects on 5-HT and NA, as well as on other neurotransmitter systems *(Table 2)*. They block muscarinic cholinergic receptors, causing constipation, blurred vision, dry mouth, and drowsiness. They block α_1 receptors, leading to postural hypotension and dizziness, and hista-

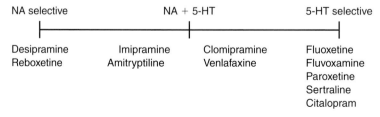

Figure 16

Effects of antidepressants on 5-HT and NA reuptake.

Table 2   Adverse effects of TCAs.

Cause	Effect
5-HT increase	Nausea, gastrointestinal and sexual dysfunction
NA increase	Tachycardia, sweating
Cholinergic blockade	Constipation, blurred vision, dry mouth, drowsiness
α_1 blockade	Postural hypotension, dizziness
Histamine blockade	Drowsiness, weight gain
Other	Epileptic seizures

mine H_1 receptors, causing drowsiness and weight gain. They are highly toxic in overdose (except lofepramine), primarily because of their cardiovascular effects.

As described above, TCAs are metabolized in the liver by the cytochrome P_{450} system. This means that drugs which inhibit this system (such as SSRIs) inhibit TCA metabolism and can produce potentially toxic drug levels with apparent therapeutic doses.

Monoamine oxidase inhibitors (MAOIs)

Although they are only very rarely used in this age group, it is important to understand the mechanism of action of monoamine oxidase inhibitors (MAOIs) for completeness.

In the CNS the monoamine neurotransmitters (5-HT, NA and DA) are primarily broken down (deaminated) by the MAO enzyme, which is found in the mitochondria of the presynaptic nerve terminal. Two subtypes of the MAO enzyme have been identified: MAO-A, which deaminates 5-HT and NA; and MAO-B, which deaminates phenylethylamine and benzylamine. DA and tyramine (present in, for example, cheese and yeast products) are destroyed by both MAO-A and MAO-B. Tyramine increases the release of NA from the terminal which in the absence of an MAOI, is then destroyed by MAO. The well-known 'cheese reaction' is explained by the intake of tyramine-containing foods in the presence of an MAOI. Tyramine still produces an increase in NA but this cannot be destroyed by MAO and a potentially dangerous increase in blood pressure results. The classical MAOIs (phenelzine, isocarboxacid and tranylcypromine) bind to both subtypes of the MAO enzyme and inactivate them, leading to an accumulation of 5-HT, NA and DA in the presynaptic nerve terminal (Figure 14). The bond between drug and enzyme is irreversible, so the effects of MAOIs continue for 2–3 weeks after the drug is withdrawn (the time it takes for new enzyme to be synthesized). Tranylcypromine has some stimulant effects because, in addition to its MAO inhibition, it has a weak releasing action on 5-HT and NA in the presynaptic nerve terminal.

Reversible inhibitor of MAO-A (RIMA)

The only RIMA available in the UK is moclobemide. This drug class has two important potential advantages over the classical MAOIs, both reflected in its name. It is selective for the MAO-A enzyme, the subtype concerned with the metabolism of 5-HT and NA, which means that the MAO-B subtype is left free to metabolize tyramine. The risk of a tyramine food reaction is therefore greatly reduced, and there is no need for a restricted diet. It also forms a reversible bond with the enzyme, so it can be displaced if large amounts of tyramine are present. Although moclobemide has been little studied in children, the adult literature suggests that it is generally better tolerated than the classical MAOIs but it has the disadvantage of seeming to be less clinically effective as an antidepressant.

Selective serotonin reuptake inhibitors (SSRIs)

As their name implies, SSRIs selectively block the reuptake of 5-HT into the presynaptic terminal by binding at 5-HT uptake sites *(Figure 14)*. Again, these effects occur within 24 h; although, as with the TCAs and probably for similar reasons, therapeutic benefits are not usually seen for 10–20 days. The increased concentration of 5-HT in the synapse acts on the postsynaptic receptors to cause the desired effect.

Although SSRIs are effective at treating a variety of disorders, there are clear differences in both their presumed mechanism of action and their clinical effects.

In depression the important area of postsynaptic neurotransmitter increase is thought to be in the prefrontal cortex, in panic disorder it appears to be the limbic system and brainstem which are important, and in OCD in the basal ganglia.

The differences between the clinical effects of SSRIs in the different conditions are summarized in *Table 3*. An exacerbation of anxiety is often produced at the start of treatment in panic disorder but not in the other conditions. This has resulted in the recommendation to use half the starting dose for the first 1–2 weeks of treatment for panic disorder. The dose typically required to achieve response is also different, with higher doses being needed for panic disorder and OCD. A similar picture is also reflected in the duration of treatment required for the different disorders, with the longest being recommended for OCD.

The effects of SSRIs on postsynaptic serotonergic receptors explain many of their side-effects (stimulation of $5-HT_2$ receptors causes agitation, sleep disruption and the sexual problems frequently reported, and stimulation of $5-HT_3$ receptors causes nausea, gastrointestinal (GI) disturbance and headache) *(Table 4)*. Of the SSRIs, fluoxetine has the most $5-HT_2$ agonist effects and is therefore most likely to cause agitation, sleep and sexual dysfunction.

Table 3 Summary of the differences in the use of SSRIs in different conditions.

	Daily dose (e.g. for paroxetine)	Anxiety exacerbation at start of treatment	Speed of response	Duration of treatment
Depression	20 mg	No	2–4 weeks	6–9 months
Panic disorder	Up to 40 mg	Yes	4–6 weeks	9–12 months
Social anxiety disorder	20 mg	No	6–12 weeks	9–12 months
OCD	Up to 60 mg	No	6–12 weeks	At least 1 year

Table 4   Adverse effects of SSRIs.

Symptom	Receptor responsible
Insomnia	$5\text{-}HT_2$
Motor activation/anxiety	$5\text{-}HT_2$
Sexual dysfunction	$5\text{-}HT_2$
Diarrhoea	$5\text{-}HT_3$
Nausea	$5\text{-}HT_3$
Headaches	$5\text{-}HT_3$

The SSRIs are generally safe and 'clean' drugs, with much more limited effects on other neurotransmitter systems than the older TCAs and MAOIs. There have been a few reports of SSRIs (e.g. paroxetine) causing akathisia and frank extrapyramidal side-effects (EPS) which may be explained by interactions between the DA and 5-HT transmitter systems.

The differences between the SSRIs are mainly due to differences in their half-lives, the presence of active metabolites, and their different propensities to inhibit the P_{450} system (and therefore the rate of inter-activity with other drugs which use this route of metabolism) (Chapter 5). *Table 5* summarizes some of these.

Because of the effects on 5-HT, there is the risk of a serotonergic syn-drome (agitation, confusion, tremor, hyperreflexia, shivering, diarrhoea, and fever) with the combination of SSRIs and other drugs that raise 5-HT levels, i.e. MAOIs or lithium. It is therefore recommended that they should not be used in combination with MAOIs at all, and only with care with lithium. Care should also be taken when switching from an SSRI to an MAOI, allowing an adequate 'washout' period of at least five half-lives, which in the case of fluoxetine is 5 weeks.

Interestingly there is no clear relationship between plasma levels of SSRIs and their clinical effect which means that blood assays provide lit-tle information and are therefore not indicated routinely.[1]

Nefazodone

Nefazodone blocks the reuptake of 5-HT (and to an extent NA) in a similar way to the SSRIs, but in addition potently blocks the postsynaptic $5\text{-}HT_2$ receptor *(Figure 17)*. This reduces $5\text{-}HT_2$ effects seen with SSRIs (i.e. sleep problems, sexual dysfunction, motor activation) and so nefazodone should probably be used when these are particularly problematic.

The side-effects of nefazodone can be understood in terms of their increasing 5-HT availability at the $5\text{-}HT_3$ receptors (GI disturbance, headache) and blocking the $5\text{-}HT_2$ receptor (e.g. sedation).

Table 5   Differences between the SSRIs and other antidepressants.

Generic name	Also known as	Dose mg/day	Formulation available	Half-life	Active metabolites	Inhibits P_{450} system
SSRIs						
Citalopram	Cipramil	20–60	T/L	36 h	Y	2D6+
Fluoxetine	Prozac	20–60	T/L	9 days	Y[a]	2D6++
Fluvoxamine	Faverin/Luvox	100–300	T	15 h	N	3A4
Paroxetine	Seroxat/Paxil	20–60	T/L	24 h	N	2D6+++
Sertraline	Lustral/Zoloft	50–150	T	26 h	N	2D6++
Nefazodone	Dutonin/Serzone	400–600	T	2–4 h	Y	3A4
Venlafaxine	Effexor	75–375	T	11 h*	Y	Weak 2D6
Moclobemide	Manerix	300–600	T	1–4 h	Y	U
Reboxetine	Edronax	4–8	T	13 h	U	U
Mirtazapine	Zispin/Remeron	15–45	T	20–40 h	Y	U

[a]Has a very long half-life (up to 20 days) – hence 5-week washout period required from the time fluoxetine is stopped before starting on other drugs which might interact, e.g. MAOIs.

T, tablet; L, liquid; +, propensity to inhibit – i.e. Paroxetine > Fluoxetine > Sertraline; U, unlikely; * slow release formulations.

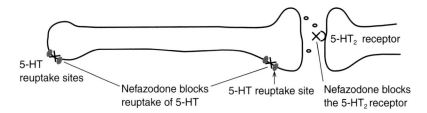

Figure 17

Site of action of nefazodone.

Selective serotonin and noradrenaline reuptake inhibitors (SNRIs)

The only SNRI currently available in the UK is venlafaxine. This works like the older TCAs in that it blocks the reuptake of both 5-HT and NA *(Figure 14)*, but has fewer effects on other neurotransmitter systems. At low doses, i.e. up to 100 mg/day, it tends to have mainly serotonergic effects and acts much like an SSRI, producing similar side-effects. At doses above this, NA effects also occur (e.g. increases in blood pressure, sweating). The fact that venlafaxine has effects on both 5-HT and NA means that it may be particularly effective in cases of severe or resistant depression. In this regard it is a considerably safer option than combining SSRIs with noradrenergic TCAs.

Noradrenaline reuptake inhibitor (NARI)

The only NARI currently available is reboxetine. This works by blocking the NA reuptake carrier in the brain and thereby increasing the concentration of NA in the synaptic cleft *(Figure 14)*. It has only been used in studies of depression in adults, where it seems to show particular benefits in terms of social functioning, i.e. on symptoms of reduced energy, interest and motivation – some of the core features of depression.

Reboxetine is also a relatively specific drug with only weak effects on 5-HT reuptake and no effects on that of DA. It also has no significant affinity for cholinergic and/or adrenergic receptors. The most commonly reported unwanted effects of reboxetine result from its central noradrenergic effects: dry mouth, constipation, insomnia, sweating, impotence and urinary hesitance. Symptomatic tachycardia can result due to increases in peripheral NA.

The metabolism of reboxetine has not been clearly determined and at the moment the manufacturers recommend that reboxetine should not be given together with drugs that inhibit the P_{450} enzyme system. Concomitant use of MAOIs and reboxetine should be avoided because of the potential risk of a tyramine effect, as should its use with ergot derivatives (in migraine treatments) because of the potential for blood pressure elevation.

Noradrenergic and specific serotonergic antidepressant (NaSSA)

Mirtazapine is the only NaSSA currently available. It evolved from the earlier antidepressant, mianserin, but has a unique mode of action. It enhances the availability of both NA and 5-HT by blocking presynaptic α_2 receptors on NA and 5-HT neurones, and in addition blocks postsynaptic 5-HT$_2$ and 5-HT$_3$ receptors *(Figure 18)*.

Blockade of α_2 autoreceptors reduces the inhibitory effects of NA and enhances NA neurotransmission. Blockade of α_2 receptors, which are also present on presynaptic 5-HT neurones, reduces the inhibitory effects of NA and enhances 5-HT release. 5-HT neurotransmission is further enhanced because 5-HT cell firing is under the control of NA. Increased NA neurotransmission allows more to act on 5-HT cell bodies (via α_1 receptors which are not blocked), facilitating their firing and subsequent release of 5-HT. Increased 5-HT release stimulates 5-HT$_1$ receptors (thought to be important for antidepressant effects). Blockade of 5-HT$_2$ and 5-HT$_3$ receptors prevents the typical serotonergic side-effects of insomnia, agitation, sexual dysfunction, and nausea.

In addition to the effects of mirtazapine on 5-HT and NA, it has also been shown to have a high affinity for histamine H$_1$ receptors. This

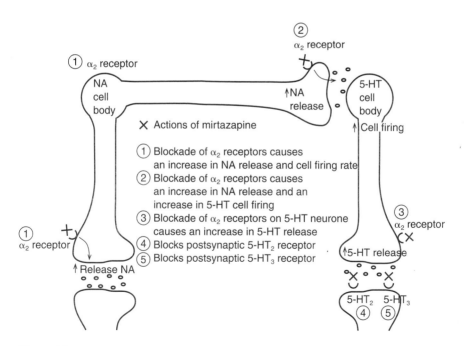

Figure 18

Mechanism of action of mirtazapine.

explains some of its most commonly reported side-effects, i.e. sedation and weight gain. Interestingly, the sedative effect of mirtazepine is greater at a low dose than at a higher; at higher doses, the increased NA offsets H_1 sedation. It also appears to be safe in overdose, with the only reports being of excessive sedation.

The available data suggest that mirtazapine has a low propensity for interactions with other drugs and is a considerably less potent inhibitor of the cytochrome P_{450} enzymes than the SSRIs fluvoxamine and fluoxetine. Like other drugs that enhance serotonergic transmission, mirtazepine should not be prescribed with, or within 14 days of stopping, an MAOI because of the risk of a serotonin syndrome.

Anxiolytics

The evolution of the currently available anxiolytics is summarized in *Figure 19*.

Benzodiazepines

Specific benzodiazepine receptors were first identified in 1977 and have now been visualized in humans using autoradiographic, SPECT and PET techniques. They have been shown to be present solely in the grey matter of the brain and to have maximal density in the cortex, cerebellum and limbic structures (especially the hippocampus and amygdala). Benzodiazepines work by binding to specific receptors on the GABA-A receptor complex (Chapter 2). They have no direct actions on the pore but exert their effects by allosterically modulating the GABA-A recognition site, thereby enhancing the actions of GABA. It is this lack of direct effects on the chloride channel that explains their safety in overdose. In contrast, the barbiturates in high doses can open the channel directly causing unchecked hyperpolarization and inhibition, resulting in severe CNS depression and subsequent death.

The GABA-A receptor complex has been cloned and found to consist of five different subunits (two α, two β, and one γ) that can be combined in a variety of ways. This allows different subtypes to exist in different parts of the CNS, although as yet the precise anatomical distribution and physiological role of each subtype remains unclear. Different subtypes show different recognition properties at the benzodiazepine-binding site and on this basis it was originally proposed that two types of benzodiazepine receptor existed (BZ_1 and BZ_2). It is now clear, however, that this is an oversimplification of the situation. This remains an important avenue for future drug development, with specific drugs being tailored to target specific receptor subtypes for particular effects (see below).

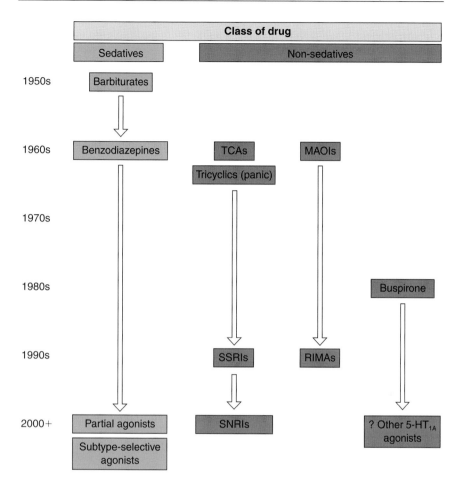

Figure 19

Evolution of anxiolytic treatment.

The benzodiazepine receptors are unique among currently known receptor systems because they exert a bidirectional effect on GABA function – agonists, inverse agonists, and antagonists all act at the same receptor. *Figure 20* shows this receptor spectrum.

Inverse agonists reduce the actions of GABA and as a result produce effects opposite to those of the agonists, i.e. are anxiogenic and convulsant. Antagonists bind to the benzodiazepine receptor and competitively block the effects of agonists and inverse agonists without having effects of their own. The first benzodiazepine antagonist to be identified was flumazenil. This has been used to treat benzodiazepine overdose and to determine whether new compounds and putative endogenous ligands act via benzodiazepine receptors. Agonists are the classical clinically useful anxiolytics, e.g. diazepam, lorazepam, chlordiazepoxide, alprazolam and clonazepam. They all enhance the actions of GABA and as a result reduce anxiety and tension, produce sedation and sleep, and possess varying degrees of muscle-relaxation and anticonvulsant properties. The side-effects they commonly cause are a consequence of this same CNS depression: sedation, ataxia, and anterograde amnesia.

The benzodiazepines have a rapid onset of action, with maximal effects being seen in the first 1–2 weeks of treatment. In this respect they compare favourably with other available anxiolytic agents, e.g. TCAs and buspirone, which both take several weeks to have effects. They are also well-tolerated in terms of reported side-effects and drop-out rates, both factors that again compare favourably with other anxiolytics, particularly the TCAs. Regarding specific symptom patterns, the benzodiazepines are particularly effective at improving sleep disturbance and in reducing somatic symptoms of anxiety, including those involving the cardiovascular and respiratory systems. There are, however, some reports of benzodiazepine-induced paradoxical agitation, excitation, and disinhibition, especially in children.

Although benzodiazepines have been used and studied extensively for more than 30 years, the optimal treatment duration for adults, let alone children, has not yet been determined. Adult guidelines have tended to emphasize short-term use only. The Royal College of Psychiatry in 1988 suggested a maximum treatment duration of 4 weeks. The American regulating body, the FDA, continues to state that the efficacy of benzodiazepines during treatments that last longer than 4 months has not been assessed by systematic studies; and the need for medication should be reassessed periodically. The lack of clarity and very conservative recommended prescribing practices derive from the two major problems asso-

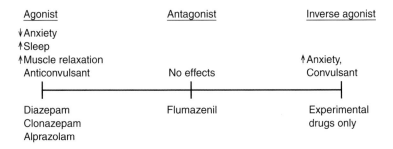

Figure 20

Agonist, antagonist and inverse agonist effects.

ciated with benzodiazepine use: tolerance and dependence. It is certainly true that for relatively short-term, stress-induced fluctuations in anxiety, and for a large proportion of chronically anxious patients, the benzodiazepines are best and most effectively used only for limited time periods. However, a certain group require treatment for considerably longer, some even on a maintenance basis. In children and adolescents the use of benzodiazepines should be confined to the acute treatment of severe anxiety or in exceptional cases where anxiety is incapacitating and unresponsive to any other approach.

5-HT$_{1A}$ agonists

Buspirone is the only 5-HT$_{1A}$ agonist available in the UK. Its mode of action is quite different from that of the benzodiazepines and related drugs in that it binds to 5-HT$_{1A}$ receptors, which are located both presynaptically (on cell bodies in the dorsal raphe) and postsynaptically *(Figure 21)*. At the cell body level, 5-HT$_{1A}$ receptors are inhibitory, decreasing presynaptic nerve firing and 5-HT release. The anxiolytic effects of buspirone are thought to be due to its actions at these cell body receptors with binding resulting in a reduction in cell firing and subsequent 5-HT release. Actions at the postsynaptic receptor may contribute to its proposed antidepressant effects.

The problems associated with buspirone are its propensity to cause nausea, headache, dizziness and nervousness at the start of treatment and, in comparison with benzodiazepines, its relatively slow onset of action *(Table 6)*. It does not, however, interact with alcohol, or cause sedation or memory impairment; and it is not associated with the problems of tolerance, dependence, and withdrawal.

Important interactions of buspirone have been reported when it is combined with other serotonergic drugs, e.g. SSRIs or MAOIs. It has also been found to cause elevations in blood pressure with MAOIs.

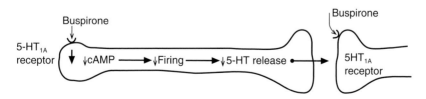

Figure 21

Sites of action of buspirone.

Table 6   Benzodiazepines versus buspirone as anxiolytic treatments.

	Advantages	Drawbacks

Benzodiazepines	Fast onset
	Early sleep
	    improvement
		Sedation
		Amnesia
		Ataxia
		Potentiates alcohol
		Abusable
		Withdrawal even
		    with low dose

Buspirone	No sedation
	No withdrawal
	No dependence
	No alcohol
	    interaction
		Slow onset
		Nausea, dizziness
		    at start

β-Blockers

β-Blockers are still widely used in the UK, particularly for anxiety symptoms, despite very limited evidence of efficacy and not insignificant risk in those with other conditions such as asthma. Their only proven role in psychiatry is for specific performance anxiety (as in musicians and actors), as a treatment for akathisia, and lithium-induced tremor. Their mechanism of action is, as the name indicates, through blockade of β-adrenergic receptors (β_1 in the CNS and heart, β_2 in blood vessels, pulmonary tree, and GI tract), which reduces NA activity.

Mood stabilizers

Several mood stabilizers with very different mechanisms of action are now available including lithium, carbamazepine, and sodium valproate. These are not only effective maintenance treatments for bipolar disorder, but are also effective in the acute treatment of manic episodes and as adjunctive treatments for resistant depression. They have also been used to alleviate symptoms in OCD, bulimia and aggression.

Lithium

The precise mechanism of action of lithium has not been clearly established. There are two main theories and both may well apply. Lithium acts predominantly through the phosphatidylinositol (PI) second messenger system to cause alterations in calcium and protein kinase C-mediated processes. It also enhances serotonergic neurotransmission through several proposed mechanisms: increasing the uptake of tryptophan into serotonergic nerves, increasing the presynaptic release of 5-HT, and upregulation of postsynaptic 5-HT_2 receptors. This may explain its efficacy in disorders associated with serotonergic abnormality, e.g. depression, and its potential to cause serotonergic syndrome (see above) when prescribed with other serotonergic agents.

The most commonly observed side-effects of lithium are gastrointestinal (nausea, diarrhoea, weight gain), polydipsia and polyuria, fine tremor, and hypothyroidism *(Table 7)*. Lithium has a narrow therapeutic window, and it is important to watch for signs of intoxication (blurred vision, increasing GI disturbance, drowsiness, coarse tremor, and ataxia), which usually require withdrawal of treatment. Signs of toxicity include hyperreflexia, convulsions, and toxic psychoses.

Carbamazepine

Carbamazepine is an anticonvulsant that is also used as a mood stabilizer. Its mechanism of action is also not clearly understood. Proposed theories include: suppression of limbic kindling; inhibition of α_2 adrenergic receptors, causing increased catecholamine release into the synaptic cleft; blockade of sodium channels, leading to an increased neuronal action potential threshold and consequently inhibitory effects; and reducing calcium influx into glial cells.

The most commonly observed side-effects of carbamazepine are shown in Table 7. Carbamazepine is also an enzyme inducer: it increases the metabolism of a variety of drugs including itself and therefore reduces their plasma levels.

Sodium valproate

Sodium valproate is also an anticonvulsant that possibly works by inhibiting key enzymes involved in GABA catabolism. This increases intracellular GABA and its release into the synaptic cleft. As described in the section on benzodiazepines, GABA induces a conformational change in the GABA-A receptor, increasing the permeability of the chloride channel

Table 7   Adverse effects of mood stabilizers.

Lithium	Tremor, sedation, GI problems, psoriasis (new or worsening), polyuria, weight gain, thyroid problems, dizziness
Carbamazepine	Ataxia, rash, dizziness
Sodium valproate	Tremor, GI problems, alopecia

and hyperpolarizing the neuronal membrane, thereby inhibiting its neuronal excitability. Sodium valproate may also suppress limbic kindling, which could explain its antimanic properties.

The most commonly observed side-effects of sodium valproate are shown in *Table 7*. Hepatotoxicity is an important but rare problem (incidence 1/120 000). The cases in which it occurred were young children (2–10 years), who usually had another neurological disorder, were on multiple anticonvulsants and were hepatitis B positive.

Antipsychotics

The discovery of neuroleptic drugs in the 1950s was one of the great breakthroughs in pharmacotherapeutics and since then more than 30 have been developed. They are, however, by no means perfect drugs and are associated with considerable side-effects.

Typical antipsychotics

All typical antipsychotics (except sulpiride, which is selective for mesolimbic/cortical D_2 receptors) block DA receptors in all the major dopaminergic pathways *(Figure 22)*. This explains both their clinical effects and their side-effect profiles. Blockade of dopaminergic neurones in the mesolimbic pathway improves psychotic symptoms. Blockade in the mesocortical pathway further decreases DA transmission there and explains the lethargy and apathy sometimes experienced. Blockade of dopaminergic projections from the substantia nigra to the basal ganglia results in well-known extrapyramidal side-effects (EPS): acute dystonia, akathisia, parkinsonian effects, and tardive dyskinesia. These are particularly likely with high-potency drugs that have significant D_2 blockade without concomitant anticholinergic capacity, e.g. haloperidol, and much less common with drugs which have substantial anticholinergic activity, e.g. thioridazine. The anticholinergic actions means that drugs with this effectively have an internal antidote to the dopaminergic blockade. Blockade of dopaminergic projections from the posterior hypothalamus to the pituitary results in increased prolactin secretion as normally this is inhibited by DA.

The clinical potency of typical antipsychotics is closely related to the affinity of the drug for the D_2 receptor, suggesting that blockade of this receptor is important for efficacy. This is not the whole story, however, because D_2 antagonism occurs almost immediately, whereas therapeutic effects are usually delayed for at least a week, suggesting that secondary changes are important. PET scans have shown that these therapeutic effects are evident if more than 70 per cent of D_2 receptors are bound by the antipsychotic and EPS occur when occupancy exceeds 80 per cent. All typical antipsychotics are equally effective, although they

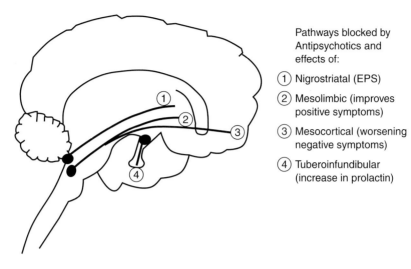

Pathways blocked by
Antipsychotics and
effects of:

(1) Nigrostriatal (EPS)

(2) Mesolimbic (improves
positive symptoms)

(3) Mesocortical (worsening
negative symptoms)

(4) Tuberoinfundibular
(increase in prolactin)

Figure 22
Effects of antipsychotics blocking all four DA pathways.

exert maximal antipsychotic effects at different doses because of differences in potency.

Most typical antipsychotics have some affinity for cholinergic, α_1-adrenergic, histaminergic, and serotonergic receptors, resulting in the expected adverse effects related to them *(Table 8)*.

Atypical antipsychotics

It was originally held that for a drug to have antipsychotic actions it must necessarily have EPS, the two being intrinsically linked. However, as the specific anatomical pathways involved became better understood, it was clear that this was not the case. The development of clozapine also challenged this original premise. In clinical studies clozapine seemed to exert selective effects on mesolimbic and mesocortical neurones rather than on striatal or tuberoinfundibular neurones, causing fewer EPS and no elevation in prolactin. It was found to be at least as effective as standard neuroleptics in terms of antipsychotic efficacy, particularly against negative symptoms, and to have superior effects in treatment-resistant patients. All these obviously represented important and desirable advances. Since then, other drugs have been developed; and specific criteria have now been elaborated to define an atypical compound. In clinical testing these include: antipsychotic efficacy; no or reduced induction of EPS and tardive dyskinesia; and no elevation of prolactin. Some researchers have also added having some efficacy on negative

Table 8   Adverse effects of typical and atypical antipsychotics.

Pharmacology	Effects
D_2 blockade in nigrostriatal pathway	EPS and tardive dyskinesia
D_2 blockade in tuberoinfundibular pathway	Hyperprolactinaemia causing galactorrhea, gynaecomastia, amennorhoea
D_2 blockade in mesocortical pathway	Production or worsening of negative symptoms
α_1 receptor blockade	Orthostatic hypotension, dizziness, sedation
Muscarinic/cholinergic receptor blockade	Dry mouth, blurred vision, constipation, impairment of cognitive function
Histaminergic receptor blockade	Weight gain, sedation
$5HT_{2C}$ receptor blockade	Weight gain, sedation

Table 9   Criteria for atypical antipsychotic.

Antipsychotic efficacy
No or reduced induction of EPS and tardive dyskinesia
No elevation of prolactin
Some efficacy on negative symptoms

symptoms as an additional criterion, although this is controversial *(Table 9)*. On the basis of these criteria in the UK, in addition to clozapine, amisulpiride, olanzapine, quetiapine, risperidone and sertindole have been labelled atypical antipsychotics.

There is no single specific receptor interaction that explains all atypical effects. Atypical antipsychotics block D_2 receptors in the mesolimbic regions, which explains their beneficial effect on positive symptoms. Some (i.e. clozapine and olanzapine) are also potent D_4 blockers. Atypical antipsychotics are also potent blockers of postsynaptic $5\text{-}HT_{2a}$ receptors. This decreases the inhibitory effects of 5-HT on dopaminergic cell firing and, as a result, causes increased dopaminergic activity, which in the prefrontal cortex may explain the often-reported improvement in negative symptoms. An alternative explanation for the effect of atypical antipsychotics is that some (clozapine, risperidone, quetiapine) also block α_2 adrenoreceptors resulting in increased noradrenaline levels in the prefrontal cortex and basal ganglia. Many atypical antipsychotics are relatively selective for the mesolimbic and mesocortical pathways compared with the nigrostriatal and tuberoinfundibular pathways, which explains their diminished potential to cause EPS or increase prolactin levels.

There is limited data on the use of atypical antipsychotics in children and adolescents except perhaps clozapine. This suggests that clozapine may be superior to the classical neuroleptics, although possibly more toxic (with an increased risk of agranulocytosis and seizures being reported).

The reader is referred to the work by Shiloh et al[2] for further reading about the areas covered in Chapters 2 and 3.

4
Mood disorders

Child psychiatrists face the increasingly complex task of deciding how best to manage children and adolescents presenting with mood disorders.

The aetiology of these conditions is multifactorial and, as evidence accumulates, it becomes apparent that they can be understood using a number of paradigms ranging from the genetic to the psychodynamic. Likewise, the modalities of treatment vary from pharmacological and physical forms to systemic, group, individual, cognitive-behavioural and interpersonal therapies. Here, we focus on understanding the mood disorders and their varied presentations in this age group from a psychopharmacological perspective and explore the various pharmacological treatments available to the clinician.

In most cases, children and adolescents presenting with mood disorders are best managed within the context of a Child and Adolescent Mental Health Service (CAMHS) multidisciplinary team setting. This allows for the careful assessment of the child's condition (which is often complex) and subsequent utilization of the team's skills to compose an optimum treatment package for the individual child and family/carers.

In the past, the notion that children and adolescents suffered from similar mood disorders to adults was controversial and contested. Research has now shown, however, that the disorders are on a continuum; and as a result they are now described in an identical way across the lifespan. What is also being increasingly recognized is that these conditions are often chronic and require lifelong monitoring for episodic recurrences, treatment and prevention. The economic implications for failing to address this are enormous, let alone the impact on the individual's personal, social and educational development and their quality of life.

Both DSM IV and ICD 10 systems classify the mood disorders in a similar way, dividing them into depressive and bipolar disorders and are applied to all ages. The depressive disorders (major depression and dysthymia) are distinguished from bipolar disorders by the fact that there is no history of ever having had a manic or hypomanic episode. We have

Table 10   DSM IV mood disorders.

Depressive disorders
    Major depressive disorder
    Dysthymic disorder (depressed mood or irritability on most days for 1 year)

Bipolar disorders
    Bipolar I disorders (manic or mixed episodes usually accompanied by one or
       more depressive episodes)
    Bipolar II disorder (major depressive episodes accompanied by at least one
       hypomanic episode)
    Cyclothymic disorder (chronic, fluctuating mood disturbance not of the severity
       of bipolar I or II for at least 1 year)

Table 11   ICD 10 mood disorders.

Recurrent depressive disorders
Bipolar affective disorder
Persistent mood (affective) disorder (cyclothymia and dysthymia)

summarized the classification here *(Tables 10 and 11)* and refer the reader to the fuller text for further details.[3,4]

These classification systems are being increasingly used in child and adolescent psychiatry and have the advantage of standardizing diagnostic processes between clinicians. There remains some uncertainty, however, about how accurately they relate to the specific field of child and adolescent psychiatry, although hopefully further work in this area will clarify the situation.

Assessment of mood disorders

The essential feature of a major depressive disorder is a clinical course characterized by one or more major depressive episodes without a history of manic or hypomanic episodes. The essential features from DSM IV are summarized below.

Symptoms of a major depressive episode

- Depressed or irritable mood
- Markedly diminished interest or pleasure in activities
- Significant weight loss or failure to make expected weight gains
- Insomnia or hypersomnia
- Psychomotor agitation or retardation
- Fatigue or loss of energy

- Feelings of worthlessness or excessive or inappropriate guilt
- Diminished ability to think or concentrate or indecisiveness
- Recurrent thoughts of death or suicide

In addition to describing the symptoms, both DSM IV and ICD 10 also specify the severity of the episode (mild, moderate, severe), the presence of psychotic symptoms, the presence of atypical features and the pattern of presentation (e.g. seasonal or rapid cycling).

Within ICD 10 there is also a separate childhood category for mixed disorders characterized by both conduct disorder and depression (depressive conduct disorder). This is an attempt to address the complexity of childhood disorders now being elucidated by research. Children with depressive conduct disorder seem to have lower rates of depressive disorder when followed up into adulthood, lower rates of depression among relatives, a worse prognosis in terms of substance abuse and greater variability of mood. For these reasons it seems that depression in conjunction with conduct disorder should be considered as a distinct disease entity.[5]

The main criteria for a diagnosis of dysthmic disorder are shown in *Table 12*.

The essential feature of a bipolar disorder is the presence of one or more hypomanic or manic episodes. A hypomanic or manic episode is a distinct period during which the predominant mood is either elevated, expansive or irritable and during which associated features also occur (summarized from DSM IV below).

Symptoms of hypomania and mania

- A distinct period of abnormally and persistently elevated, expansive or unstable mood for at least 4 days (hypomania) or 1 week (mania)
- Inflated self-esteem or grandiosity
- Decreased need to sleep
- More talkative than usual or pressure to keep talking
- Flight of ideas or subjective experience that thoughts are racing

Table 12   Diagnostic criteria for dysthymic disorder

- Depressed mood or irritability for most of the day, for most days, or for at least one year
- When depressed, presence of at least two of the following: poor appetite or overeating; insomnia or hypersomnia; low energy or fatigue; low self-esteem; poor concentration; feelings of hopelessness
- During the 1 year period the young person has never been without the symptoms above for more than 2 months at a time
- Disturbance is not accounted for by major depressive disorder

- Distractibility
- Decrease in goal-directed activity or psychomotor agitation
- Excessive involvement in pleasurable activities that have a high potential for painful consequences, such as increased risk-taking and sexual promiscuity

These episodes usually begin suddenly with a rapid escalation of symptoms over a few days and are typically briefer and end more abruptly than depressive episodes. In contrast to a manic episode a hypomanic episode is devoid of psychotic features and is not severe enough to cause a marked impairment in social functioning or hospitalization.

Identifying mood disorders in youngsters requires specialist training. They can present in a variety of ways, e.g. social withdrawal, school failure, impaired relationships and self-harm, or with disorders of behaviour or conduct.

It is also important to be aware that the symptoms reported often vary with age. Younger children with depression typically show behavioural problems including withdrawal, irritability, and apathy. They also display a range of extreme emotions such as persistent distress and crying, depressed mood and lack of enjoyment. Adolescents often describe the mood symptoms seen in adults or those associated with an 'atypical presentation' with, for example, hyperphagia, hypersomnia and excessive tiredness.

It is important to explore depressive symptomatology carefully, as this can elicit features of a disorder previously masked. The overlap between depression and other psychiatric disorders such as conduct disorder, hyperactivity, anorexia nervosa, and anxiety states is a consistent finding. Learning problems and school refusal may also coexist. It is well known that somatic complaints may hide underlying depression, but it should be remembered that medical conditions can lead to secondary depression.

With bipolar disorders, there are some similarities between mania and hypomania and overactivity, although, in the latter case, the activity tends to be less goal-directed. In older children (9–12 years), aberrations in thought content, such as grandiosity and paranoia, are common. Irritability and emotional lability are more usual in younger children. Hyperactivity, pressure of speech and distractibility occur more frequently in both age groups; and delusions and hallucinations may be present. Strober[6] suggested that prepubertal bipolar children have an illness characterized by frequent cycles of brief duration in which dysphoria and hypomania are intermixed; with the onset of puberty the cyclical extremes of depression and mania start to occur.

The assessment of mood disorders in this age group requires information from a variety of sources. Children may be able to describe subjective symptoms such as sadness, guilt, worthlessness and suicidal ideas, but parents are usually more able to report on observable changes such as sleep or appetite disruption, irritability and withdrawal. It is also very important to determine the child or adolescent's functioning within the family, peer and school setting.

Prevalence of mood disorders

It is difficult to quote figures with certainty because of the different ways in which the mood disorders have been conceptualized and measured in the past. Nevertheless, with the use of more consistent diagnostic criteria, rates of 0.5–2.5 per cent for major depression among preadolescents have recently been quoted.[7-9] Rates for adolescents are higher, at 2.0–8.0 per cent,[10] confirming the finding of increased prevalence with age. The sex ratio overall is equal or with a male predominance among preadolescents, which changes with the onset of adolescence to follow the adult pattern of female preponderance. It has been suggested that major depression is becoming more common among both adults and children.

It is estimated that the lifetime prevalence of bipolar disorder is 0.4–1.6 per cent. Approximately 10–15 per cent of adolescents with recurrent major depressive episodes will go on to develop bipolar disorder. Recent epidemiological studies show that, unlike major depressive disorder, bipolar disorder has an equal sex ratio.

Long-term studies on mood disorders show that they are chronic disorders with episodes recurring throughout the lifespan. In adolescents, the rate of recurrence may be more frequent than that reported in adults, with more than 40 per cent having a repeat episode within 1 year.

Suicide

Suicide in preadolescent children is rare but increases for both genders in the adolescent years.[11] The suicide rate among young males is increasing with the consequence that suicide is now the second most common cause of death among young people aged 15–24 years.[12] The new difference is shown by the 1990 suicide rates per million in England and Wales for males and females aged 15–19 years which were 57 and 14 respectively.[11] Mental illness and suicide specifically have been targeted as part of the Health of the Nation's drive to reduce fatality rates. Questions have been raised about the underlying cause of death from accidents or other risk-taking activities in this age group and whether the increased prevalence of mood disorders may account for the apparent rise in the suicide rate; an important point given the potential treatability of mood disorders. Characteristics that seem to distinguish depressed children or adolescents who make a suicide attempt from those who do not, include cognitive distortions, life stressors, hopelessness, impulsivity, and inability to tolerate intense negative affect or emotional distress and anger.[13] Further research into such factors will hopefully inform the debate.

Comorbidity

Coexistence of mood disorders with other conditions is a consistent finding, the most common being shown below. Interestingly, adolescents with depressive disorders seem to be more likely to have an additional psychiatric condition than depressed adults.

Common comorbid disorders

- Anxiety disorders
- Conduct disorders
- Hyperactivity
- Anorexia nervosa
- School refusal
- Substance misuse (alcohol, cocaine, cannabis, etc.)
- Somatic complaints (e.g. abdominal pain)
- Other medical conditions (e.g. diabetes, cystic fibrosis, inflammatory bowel disease)

Aetiology of mood disorders

Neurochemical theories

The catecholamine theory of affective disorders, stating that depression was associated with a deficit of NA neurotransmission and mania with an excess, was first published by Schildkraut[14] and later expanded to include an abnormality of serotonergic function. This view of neurotransmitter functioning is, however, too simplistic and has been challenged by several observations, particularly the well-known finding of the clinical response of antidepressants being delayed for 2–3 weeks despite the fact that synaptic monoamine changes occur within 24 hours. Current theories of monoamine abnormalities in mood disorders now address both monoamine activity in the synapse and receptor/second messenger abnormalities.

5-HT abnormalities

A decrease in serotonergic function has been implicated in the pathology of the mood disorders although the precise location of the deficit has not been established.

5-HT metabolites
Cerebrospinal fluid (CSF) levels of 5-HIAA (the breakdown product of 5-HT) are used as an indirect measure of central serotonergic activity. Some studies have reported lower levels in depressed patients although it appears that low CSF 5-HIAA is most consistently linked with higher violent suicide risk rather than depression itself. Lower levels of tryptophan, 5-HT and 5-HIAA have also been found in the postmortem brains of depressed suicide victims compared with non-depressed subjects.

Depletion studies
5-HT can be reduced by depleting subjects of the 5-HT precursor tryptophan. When this has been done in adults who have responded to treatment with serotonergic antidepressants they become acutely depressed, a state that lasts for a few hours until normal tryptophan levels are restored.[15] This suggests that the availability of 5-HT in the synapse is crucial for antidepressant response.

Platelet studies
Platelets are considered to be a model for central 5-HT neurones and studies of these have shown that the rate of 5-HT uptake and the number of [^{3}H]imipramine binding sites are reduced in patients with depression.

Receptor binding
There appears to be reduced $5\text{-}HT_{1A}$ and increased $5\text{-}HT_2$ receptor function in depression. The evidence for reduced $5\text{-}HT_{1A}$ function comes from postmortem studies of receptor numbers and results from challenge studies showing blunted $5\text{-}HT_{1A}$ effects. Increased $5\text{-}HT_2$ receptor binding has been found in the prefrontal cortex of postmortem brains of depressed suicide victims. Similarly increased $5\text{-}HT_2$ receptor binding has been found in platelets from subjects with major depression and neuroendocrine effects which are mediated by $5\text{-}HT_2$ receptors are also found to be increased.

   Chronic antidepressant treatment appears to upregulate postsynaptic $5\text{-}HT_{1A}$ receptors and downregulate $5\text{-}HT_2$ receptors. The effects of antidepressants on $5\text{-}HT_{1A}$ presynaptic receptors are described in Chapter 2.

NA abnormalities

Evidence for a dysfunctional NA system comes from a variety of sources, but almost exclusively adult studies.

Metabolites
Plasma and urinary measures of MHPG are consistently lower in bipolar and unipolar depressives compared with normal controls.

Depletion studies

When reserpine (which depletes presynaptic catecholamine stores) was used as an antihypertensive treatment, it was found to produce symptoms of depression suggesting that depleting presynaptic NA levels produced depression. More recent studies with α-methylparatyrosine (an inhibitor of NA metabolism) have reported similar results to those seen with tryptophan depletion, i.e. a transient but rapid mood lowering particularly in patients who had responded to NA antidepressants.

Platelet studies

Platelet studies suggest reduced α_2 receptor binding in depression.

Receptor binding

Abnormalities of both α- and β-adrenergic receptors have been implicated in depression. There is evidence of reduced postsynaptic α_2 function in depression, with a blunted growth hormone response to clonidine, an α_2 agonist. There have been reports of increased α_2 and β-receptor binding in patients who have committed suicide.

Binding studies show that antidepressant treatment downregulates presynaptic α_2 and postsynaptic β receptors.

Summary of proposed neurotransmitter changes with antidepressant treatment

There is evidence of reduced synaptic availability of 5-HT and NA in depression which may lead to a compensatory increase in postsynaptic receptor function or number. Over the course of several weeks of antidepressant treatment, presynaptic receptors desensitize, resulting in reduced inhibition of cell firing and an increase in neurotransmitter release in the synapse. This may then lead to a compensatory downregulation of some postsynaptic receptors, e.g. 5-HT$_2$ and β receptors.

It should be remembered that very few of these studies have been performed in children and adolescents and, as a result, theories from adult populations have been extrapolated to explain the disorders.

The developmental aspects of psychobiological responses have not been clearly elucidated. The increased rates of mood disorders in adolescence may well be attributable to the biological or hormonal changes (or both) which occur at puberty. The precise reasons are at present unclear although hormone status appears to be particularly important. For example, it is known that oestrogen is selectively taken up by aminergic neurones in the brain and may regulate their function. Progesterone metabolites, made in the brain, have recently been shown to modulate GABA function.

Neuroanatomical

Structural changes found in mood disorders using computed tomography (CT) and magnetic resonance imaging (MRI) are similar in adults and children/adolescents. The main findings indicate a decrease in frontal lobe volume and an increase in ventricular volume in depressed (both unipolar and bipolar) subjects compared to normal controls. The frontal lobe (and prefrontal cortex in particular) is known to play an important role in cognitive functioning and has inputs from both 5-HT and NA systems.

Functional studies using single photon emission tomography (SPECT) and positron emission tomography (PET) provide a useful means of examining brain function through measures of cerebral bloodflow and cerebral metabolic rate. There have been more than 100 such studies in adult major depressive and bipolar disorder. These show evidence of decreased bloodflow in the prefrontal cortex and basal ganglia with possible involvement of regions of the limbic system.[16] There have been far fewer studies in children and adolescents but those that there have been have confirmed the findings of the adult studies.[16,17] It is possible that decreased perfusion of the frontal cortex might account for the impulsivity and diminished sense of self-control with the subsequent increase in suicide rates seen in mood disorders.

Genetic factors

Twin and adoption studies in the adult literature support a strong genetic link for unipolar (monozygotic/dizygotic 54% : 20%) and bipolar (monozygotic/dizygotic 79% : 19%) disorders. The lifetime prevalence of depressive disorder in the relatives of depressed children have been shown to be double that found in the relatives of closely matched non-depressed controls.[18] Evidence suggests that early-onset disorders among children have a genetic loading. It also appears clinically that those children who have a strong genetic loading for depressive disorder exhibit symptoms at a younger age which are possibly also of a more severe nature.

Goodyer et al.[19] discussed how families of depressed adolescent girls seemed to become more 'life event prone' as a result of parental psychopathology. This clearly raises a debate regarding the significance of genetic versus environmental causality and suggests that an interactive model is the most plausible.

Sleep and depression

The classic abnormalities of sleep found in depression include the clinical observations of difficulty getting off to sleep, waking during the night and early-morning waking. The main objective findings are decreased

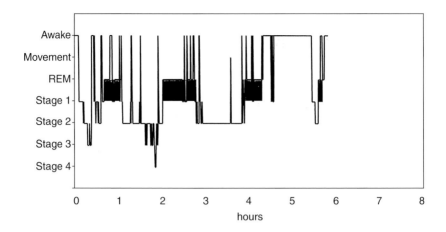

Figure 23

Sleep changes seen in depression.

REM latency, an increased amount of REM sleep and reduced slow wave sleep early in the night *(Figure 23)*. Studies in children and adolescents show similar findings to those in the adult literature and provide further evidence of the biological nature of major depression.

Psychological mechanisms

Understanding how those suffering from mood disorders think and feel has led to the development of psychological theories to explain some of the links.

Seligman's classic work on rats[20] proposed the model of 'learned helplessness'. These studies described a posture that rats took when repeatedly exposed to traumatic physical experiences and which they developed when re-exposed to such threats. From this it was hypothesized that a depressed person succumbs to negative experiences (e.g. physical/emotional/sexual abuse) and gives up the will to care or respond.

The most persuasive psychological view of depression was proposed by Beck and colleagues[21] who described the self-defeating cognitions frequently seen in depression as a triad of negative thoughts relating to the self, the world, and the future. They explained how negative automatic thoughts lead a person into the depths of despair and depression. Cognitive therapy developed from this theory. During treatment the negative automatic thoughts are identified and challenged and strategies developed to counteract them.

Adolescents are particularly susceptible to changes in their peer relationships. Vulnerable youngsters from at-risk families can respond adversely to rejection from their peers, further lowering their self-confidence and potentially leading to depression. Understanding the developmental aspects of adolescence and questioning the basis of adolescent turmoil have raised the issue of whether some adolescents are actually experiencing depressive episodes. Some may attempt, consciously or otherwise, to self-medicate by misusing alcohol and drugs, some engage in other high-risk activity and others commit suicide.

Psychosocial

Understanding the influence of psychosocial factors on the child is a complex task. Visualizing systems *(Figure 24)* helps us to understand the child's difficulties within the context of their family and environment over time. This allows us to look at the interactive nature of adversity and highlights how difficulty in one area can have a direct influence on another.

It has been clearly established that parental mood disorders can have a direct impact on a child's environment. Mother–child interactions reduce and are more hostile in nature, so creating a stressful environment for the child. Reduced mother–child interactions and maternal distress can create a vicious cycle of tense interpersonal relationships and subsequent behavioural difficulties within the child. There may also be an association with family discord[22] and marital difficulties which ultimately lead to separation and divorce – a further loss, although some studies suggest that the final reduction of family discord within the home is more beneficial for the child.

It is important to consider a variety of factors and how they combine and impact on the individual child and their family *(Table 13)*. These need to be considered alongside a detailed chronology of the child's

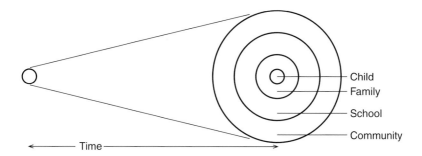

Figure 24
Psychosocial systems.

Table 13

Life events
    Loss and bereavement
    Divorce and separation
    Trauma – physical/emotional/sexual abuse/disasters
    Ill-health

Chronic adversity
    Family and marital discord
    Domestic violence
    Physical/emotional deprivation
    Socio-economic adversity
    Periods in local authority care

Vulnerability factors
    Genetic susceptibility to mental illness
    Substance misuse
    Learning disability
    Adverse temperament
    Negative attributional style of thinking

Resilience/protective factors
    Availabililty of a confiding adult
    Supportive peer relationships
    Likeable characteristics/temperament of the child
    Educational/occupational/family attainment

development, attachments and relationships within the context of their family and community.

Assessment and treatment

General clinical principles for starting treatment

The cornerstone of good clinical practice is a thorough assessment of the child's presenting difficulties and their associated history within the context of the child's and family's psychosocial environment. The child and adolescent psychiatrists' training allows the clinician to use an eclectic approach while relying on their medical training, their knowledge of the psychological theories (systemic, psychodynamic, learning and cognitive) and their experience of paediatric and adult psychiatry to help them illicit an in-depth understanding of the issues. Drawing on the multidisciplinary expertise of the CAMHS team members allows us to be trained in completing a comprehensive assessment, although the child psychiatrist per se oversees the prescription of medication. The opportunity for such specialist training for paediatricians may be a development for the future.

This is by no means an over inclusive account of such an assessment but it offers the reader a flavour of the difference between an adult psychiatry interview and that routinely carried out within a child and family clinic setting.

Ideally the whole household would be invited to the initial assessment appointment and a note made of who attends. Obviously the form of presentation will determine the focus and order of events covered. For example, a clinician undertaking a routine request from a general practitioner for an assessment of a 7-year old will have different initial priorities to a clinician carrying out a deliberate self-harm assessment of a 16-year old admitted to the ward following a paracetemol overdose. However, in both instances, a full and detailed history will inform the optimum management plan.

It is worth outlining at the start that the clinician wishes to hear everybody's personal view of the present difficulties and that they would expect that there would be some similarities and differences expressed. It is often informative to have an understanding of the individual expectations of the family members about the appointment and their view about the potential outcome of the session.

The art of successful history taking rests in engaging the youngster and family in a joint therapeutic alliance in which opinions are respected and concerns shared. An opportunity for the child or adolescent to be seen separately from the main carers should be offered, alongside time for the parents to be seen together, or sometimes separately if for example there is an acrimonious parental separation. Similar space should be allowed in the case of professional child carers. This allows the clinician to observe how the youngster and carers manage this separation and reunion, and gauge whether the response is appropriate given the developmental level of the young person.

Information regarding the present symptomatology needs to be explored in some detail to ascertain the onset of the difficulties and its relationship to any significant changes, life events or stresses within the family or environment. Following an episode of deliberate self-harm there is a more specific focus which needs to be systematically relived in order to understand the cognitions of the child at the time and how they appear after the event. The question 'Why?' needs to be routinely asked in addition to identifying what has changed to make a repeat episode less likely. More sinister signs of there having been some contemplation, planning with serious intent, the presence of a suicidal note, attempts to prevent exposure, lack of remorse or persistent feelings of hopelessness are all of particular concern. Details regarding the form of self-harm, whether cutting to express release of pent-up feelings or more violent means of strangulation or hanging to end their distress, need to be explored. Children need to be asked what they thought would happen if they used a certain method or if they took certain pills, as medically non-toxic medication may be perceived by a child to be life threatening, and highlights the need to take any form of self-harm seriously.

An assessment of the child's understanding of death given their cognitive level needs to be elucidated, and clinicians should accept that young children can contemplate suicide as a means of escaping their distress. Unfortunately despite the rarity of such events a youngster, especially if male, is more likely to engage in an impulsive act such as strangulation or hanging, and this may end in a fatality when perhaps their intent was to escape a situation in which their experience of intense negative affect was intolerable. Fortunately prompt medical attention can be life saving. If the young person does not perceive their situation to have changed after the event the likelihood of repetition is higher.

The presence and duration of manic symptomatology should be specifically sought including evidence of atypical features. In younger children thoughts, feelings and emotions related to sadness may be more prevalent and more evident by observational changes in behaviour noted by carers and other professionals.

Various clinical techniques can be used to help a child or adolescent who has regressed to an earlier, perhaps even preverbal stage, to communicate. Examples of the youngster's play, art, or writing can be informative in assessing their preoccupations and negative cognitions. Collateral reports from significant others and teaching staff are invaluable.

Enlisting the help of siblings to give an account of their concerns about the index child can often raise the self-esteem of an otherwise dejected child who has come to believe that nobody cares. Frequently the assessment is the first forum for emotionally deprived or violent families to have an opportunity to hear their children's views, and this can be very empowering for a distressed child and their family. On other occasions intense negative emotion needs to be expressed but managed by the clinician, especially if it is clearly abusive.

The first part of the interview therefore allows for considerable information to be gleaned regarding the emotional state of the individual members including an assessment of the parents' mental state, their own stage of psychological development, their emotional availability and their capacity to appropriately parent their children and meet their needs within the clinical setting.

Having established a clear description of the quality of the child's attachments to others, a systematic appraisal of their early developmental milestones needs to be made. A three-generational genogram sets the scene and outlines significant additions and losses in the family. Details of past family psychiatric history and its treatment are invaluable.

Questions about the youngsters first few months of life can often lighten a tense situation especially if the account to date has been particularly negative.

Evidence for disorders of attachment or maternal depression or anxiety may come to light, especially if the narrative regarding early details is incoherent or the mother has difficulty recalling information. The parental adaptation to and readiness for parenthood, the partner's role and the effect of children on the marital relationship and extended family can be informative. The male may perceive an acute sense of rejection from the partner with the arrival of new or subsequent children, which can have an impact on relationships, and the psychological development of the child. The ability of siblings to tolerate change and manage angry emotions conscious or otherwise and the parental capacity to facilitate its healthy resolution can be ascertained.

Details regarding maternal well-being (both during pregnancy and perinatally), the form and ease of delivery, and the well-being of the infant including the presence of obstetric or neonatal complications are useful. This helps to give a wider perspective to the assessment especially if there is evidence of developmental disorders during the early years. A systematic chronology of the physical, emotional, psychological and social milestones will reveal features of any comorbid disorders and any areas of abnormality can be followed up with more specific questions.

Specific details about the child's temperament and his/her ability to manage emotions as an infant is often telling. The parents' capacity to facilitate the optimal level of development during the early years is considered. This can once again become an issue in relation to care and control during adolescence, especially if the parents have not successfully negotiated their own stage of adolescent development. Apparently normal development in other siblings may indicate more individual issues for the index child or point to interpersonal difficulties with certain family members. The quality and consistency of early care and whether the youngster experienced unconditional love and attention from trusted adults or not is significant.

An account of the child's ability to separate and relate to peers, their ability to successfully manage new situations including the commencement of playgroup, nursery and school should also include an assessment of the parents' readiness for these events. An outline of the child's school life, positive attributes, interests and difficulties including the qualities of their relationships with those in authority is useful.

The time of secondary transfer can often be traumatic for those with low self-esteem or vulnerability to mood disorders, as the development of new relationships can be too challenging and lead to isolation. Likewise the increase in academic demands can uncover scholastic difficulties then or indeed earlier in school life and create secondary difficulties. Unidentified disorders can result in bullying and associated problems such as anxiety, school refusal or truancy. Their ability to negotiate the developmental challenges of adolescence, sexual maturity, separation and identity will be dependent on a number of genetic and environmental factors. The onset of a formal disorder at this stage may be evident by the inability of the adolescent to make the expected progress in a number of areas of development while the family inadvertently collude. Secondary difficulties such as drug and alcohol misuse may be an attempt conscious or otherwise for the youngster to self medicate or act out their distress. An adapted mental state examination is conducted for completeness.

Baseline measures of functioning are useful. These include the use of self-rating scales such as the Beck Depression Inventory and the Mania Rating Scale, which gauge the subjective severity of depressive and manic symptoms respectively and monitor change over time. Global functioning can be assessed and reassessed using the Global Assessment Scale of the Diagnostic and Statistical Manual of Mental Disorders,[3] which can be completed by various informants.

It is also important to perform a physical examination before treatment, including recording a measure of height, weight and blood pressure (sitting and standing), as well as baseline blood investigations, such as full blood count (FBC), erythrocyte sedimentation rate (ESR), C reactive protein (CRP), urea and electrolytes (U&Es), liver function tests (LFTs) and thyroid function tests (TFTs). This not only helps to rule out comorbid disorders but also allows the clinician to detect iatrogenic haematological or biochemical abnormalities, should they arise.

By taking this form of developmental history and examination the clinician will be able to reach a formulation which leads to a diagnosis with a clear idea of the predisposing, precipitating and perpetuating factors alongside an understanding of the intergenerational issues and the ability of the youngster and their family to engage in a tailored management plan.

Having made the diagnosis, the young person and family need to be informed about the condition and the factors that play a part in its aetiology and maintenance. Information regarding the natural history and course of the disorder, the risks and benefits associated with the various treatment options and the expected length of treatment should be discussed, together with the good news that treatment reduces the severity and duration of the disorder. During the course of this discussion parents sometimes express concerns about the use of psychotropic medication. It is best to be open and honest about the present evidence to support the efficacy in the adult population and the increasing clinical experience of the benefit of some types of medication in adolescence. The need to use medication in younger children (8–11 years) is appropriately restricted to severe disorders. Although rare, fortunately positive results have been noted. Over the period of treatment parents usually see the benefits for themselves. Information sheets about the medication and potential side-effects are helpful. A simple explanation of the mechanism of action of the drug on neurotransmitters and receptors in the brain as well as other parts of the body (hence the side-effects) often helps. It is important to emphasize the fact that there is often a time lag between taking medication and the experience of benefits. This prevents unrealistic expectations which can lead to the medication being stopped prematurely, as it is perceived to be not working. It should also be explained that the medication needs to be taken regularly, ideally at the same time of day, to build up to a therapeutic level. Where appropriate, warnings about interactions with other drugs, including alcohol and over-the-counter medications, should be given. It is often helpful to record side-effects. A baseline rating helps to elicit those features which are part of the illness rather than related to the drug. Visits to the prescribing clinician need to be frequent to allow regular review of the youngster's mental state, including their suicidal risk, and the gradual adjustment of medication according to their progress. Medication should usually only be prescribed at 2-weekly intervals and it is good practice to ask a parent or guardian to oversee its administration. Both these approaches improve compliance and help to minimize the risk of an overdose. In the event of an overdose or other suicide attempt being made, swift medical attention should be sought with admission to a paediatric ward for treatment and observation.

Significantly this assessment process is therapeutic in its own right. Often two or three sessions can be enough to allow the family and young person to reach a level of understanding which helps them to effect positive change. Identifying the salient issues and providing the appropriate level of support in the problem areas can result in progress. This is more likely to be the case if the mood disorder is mild to moderate or reactive in nature and the family has the capacity to think psychologically. However, if the concerns are deemed by the clinician to be serious and the youngster is suicidal, engagement and containment in its own right may not be enough. The authors believe that this is when serious consideration needs to be given to contemplating a pharmacological approach. For a major depressive episode an SSRI is the first line of treatment. If despite an adequate therapeutic trial this fails switching to an SNRI is warranted. Augmentation strategies as outlined later should be considered while lithium should be considered for a bipolar disorder. Medication can alter the youngster's mood enough to allow them to become more available and able to use psychological treatment. This should always be offered alongside pharmacological treatment while the timing, intensity, quality and form of the intervention should be finely tuned to the individual needs of each family.

Antidepressants – the research findings

As described in Chapter 2, the antidepressants available to the clinician include MAOIs and RIMAs, TCAs, SSRIs, nefazadone, the SNRI venlafaxine, reboxetine and mirtazapine. Studies of the use of these drugs in children and adolescents with major depression are, however, very limited. This section describes the few trials that there have been, with emphasis being given to randomized, double-blind placebo-controlled studies.

TCAs

Tricyclic antidepressants have unproven efficacy in major depression in children and adolescents.[23–26] Open studies produced response rates of 75 per cent but controlled trials showed that TCAs were no more effective than placebo. This is markedly different from the response seen in adult studies where TCAs are seen to be equally effective as other antidepressants (although more toxic), typically producing improvement in 60–70 per cent of patients. Reasons for this lack of efficacy are not clear but may include the fact that TCAs also block postsynaptic receptors of other neurotransmitter systems. These receptors may be particularly sensitive in children and adolescents and may therefore interfere with the therapeutic action of TCAs. The lack of efficacy of TCAs, combined with their adverse side effect profile of neuro and cardiac toxicity, especially in overdose, as well as reports of sudden death,[27] makes the use of TCAs in this age group almost obsolete.

SSRIs

As described before, although studies with depressed children and adolescents are limited, there is accumulating evidence that the SSRIs are effective in major depression in this age group, with response rates being more similar to those seen in adults. The available data suggest that they are safe, at least in the short term, although further research is needed to provide information about their use in the long term in this age group.[28,29]

The trials are summarized below for each SSRI.

Two double-blind placebo-controlled studies have examined the use of fluoxetine in depression, one in the age group 7–17 years,[30] and one in adolescents aged 13–18 years.[31] In the first study, 96 children and adolescents were treated with fluoxetine 20 mg/day or placebo for 8 weeks. Results showed that 56 per cent of the patients on fluoxetine responded, compared with 33 per cent of the patients on placebo. Interestingly the data were analysed to try and identify potential predictors of response, but none were found.[32] In the second study, 32 adolescents were treated with doses up to 60 mg/day for 8 weeks. Although there were improvements in all symptoms apart from sleep with fluoxetine, overall there were no significant differences between the SSRI and placebo groups. Evidence from open trials with doses of fluoxetine ranging from 10 to 60 mg/day have typically shown response rates of 70–80 per cent (summarized in Bostic et al 1999).[33]

One multisite controlled study has been conducted with paroxetine (mean dose 28 mg/day) in 275 adolescents aged 12–19 years, in which it was compared with imipramine and placebo. This produced response rates of 66 per cent for paroxetine, 57 per cent for imipramine and 43 per cent for placebo, with significantly more patients reporting adverse events with imipramine leading to their discontinuation from the study.[34] Although these results are promising, the fact that this study has never been published in a peer-reviewed journal raises some questions over its validity. Two open-label studies of paroxetine in adolescents[35] and patients <14 years old[36] produced response rates of 76 and 100 per cent, respectively.

There have been no controlled studies of children or adolescents with depression using sertraline. Three open-label studies have been conducted using doses of 25–200 mg/day. One study,[37] involving 13 patients aged 12–18 years, showed a continued improvement in symptoms after 12 weeks of treatment. Another,[38] on patients aged 8–18 years, showed that 65 per cent of patients improved with older patients seeming to benefit most. The third[39] described 53 adolescents with major depressive disorder who were treated with sertraline. By 10 weeks a maximal response was obtained and included significant improvement differences from baseline rating scales. The improvement proved to be maintained with medication for 22 weeks.

There have also been no controlled studies in depression in children and adolescents using fluvoxamine. One open-label study over 8 weeks[40] in 20 adolescents (13–17 years) receiving doses of fluvoxamine of 100–300 mg/day reported similar response rates to the other SSRIs, i.e. 66 per cent.[41]

There have been no controlled or open studies using citalopram in depression in this age group.

The adverse reactions associated with the SSRIs from these studies in children and adolescents are comparable with those seen in adults. Those most commonly reported included motor restlessness, insomnia, GI disturbance, and behavioural disinhibition or a subjective sensation of excitation. There have been a few isolated reports of hypomanic symptoms developing over the course of treatment with fluoxetine and sertraline.[42] Unfortunately, at the moment it is not possible to predict who this will occur in, but clinical characteristics suggestive of risk include depression with psychotic features, comorbid attention deficit hyper-activity disorder (ADHD) or obsessive compulsive disorder (OCD), and a personal or family history of bipolar disorder.[43] There has been some concern about suicidal ideation developing as a result of fluoxetine treatment, but this has only been seen in one study,[44] in which it was reported in 6 of 42 patients. This should not, however, be seen as typical. No other studies have confirmed this finding, but such events need to be monitored and assessed as to whether they are iatrogenic or part of the illness process.

Nefazadone
There have been no controlled trials using nefazodone in the treatment of major depression in this age group. One small open study in 10 adolescents[45] over 8 weeks produced response rates of 70 per cent with doses of less than or up to 400 mg/day.

Venlafaxine

There has been only one controlled study in major depression using ven-lafaxine. This was over 6 weeks in patients aged between 8 and 17 years.[46] Low doses were used, i.e. only 37.5 mg/day for children and 75 mg/day for adolescents, and in both drug and placebo groups weekly psychotherapy was given. Over time a significant improvement was noted although there was no difference between the drug and placebo groups. This may be explained by either the low doses used, the short duration of treatment or the effect of psychotherapy.

Reboxetine and mirtazapine

No studies have been performed using reboxetine or mirtazapine in the treatment of child and adolescent major depression.

MAOIs

While the MAOIs have been helpful in the past, particularly in adult patients reporting atypical symptoms, the fact that they necessitate adherence to a strict diet (which is difficult to implement) means that they do not have a place in the current pharmacotherapy of depression in this age group. Although RIMAs, e.g. moclobemide, offer a possible alternative approach, they have not been systematically studied in children and adolescents.

Choosing an antidepressant

There are an ever-increasing number of antidepressants for the clinician to choose from and making the right choice may seem a daunting task. The factors that need to be considered are shown in *Table 14*.

Which drug is going to work

Although about 60 per cent of children and adolescents will respond to first-line antidepressants, it would seem sensible to try and choose one which has the highest likelihood of working.

One of the clearest indicators is a previous drug response – if a partic-ular antidepressant has worked before, it is likely to do so again.

Where there is no previous history, the evidence suggests using one of the newer antidepressants; for example, an SSRI.

In cases of severe or retarded depression, the evidence from the adult

Table 14   Factors to consider in choosing an antidepressant.

Which drug is going to work?
Presence of a comorbid medical condition
Potential drug interactions
Likely side-effects
Formulation available

literature suggests that antidepressants with effects on both 5-HT and NA, e.g. venlafaxine, are the most effective, and it is probably sensible to follow this approach for similar cases in child and adolescent psychiatry.

Where depression coexists with other symptoms or disorders, e.g. panic or obsessional features, the best choice is an antidepressant which is effective for both, e.g. an SSRI *(Table 15)*.

Presence of a comorbid medical condition

Coexistent medical conditions can present problems in selecting an anti-depressant which does not worsen the physical complaint. Most antidepressants (except MAOIs and probably RIMAs, e.g. moclobemide) lower the threshold at which seizures occur, which means that using an antidepressant in a child with epilepsy is problematic but not impossible provided appropriate monitoring of the epilepsy is performed. In children already taking drugs which cause nausea, e.g. chemotherapy, SSRIs may considerably worsen this. In such cases mirtazepine (which blocks 5HTs induced nausea) may be useful.

Potential drug interactions

It is important to consider the risk of a drug–drug interaction which can lead to potentially toxic drug levels being produced. This can occur when drugs are intentionally combined or when antidepressants are changed without a washout period between them (for example, fluoxetine requires a washout period of 5 weeks to ensure that it and its active metabolites are out of the system). The interaction occurs because of the effects of medication on the P450 system. An important clinical example of this occurs with the combination of SSRIs and TCAs. SSRIs inhibit the P450 2D6 enzyme system (particularly paroxetine, fluoxetine and sertraline), which metabolizes TCAs (see Chapter 3). This means that potentially toxic TCA levels may be produced by the combination. Interactions can also occur because of effects on the same neurotransmitter producing

Table 15   Anecdotal advice re choice of SSRI/SNCI

Moderate depression	Sertraline
Severe or resistant depression	Venlafaxine
Depression and OCD	Fluvoxamine/sertraline
Depression and other anxiety disorders	Fluvoxamine/sertraline
Depression with marked loss of appetite/anorexia	Citalopram

- Avoid paroxetine if there is evidence of any neurodevelopmental disorder as extrapyramidal effects are more common
- Tend not to use fluoxetine because of the long washout period of five weeks (especially important if the antidepressant needs to be changed)

effectively an overstimulation of the system, e.g. the serotonin syndrome with serotonergic drugs (e.g. SSRIs with lithium).

Likely side-effects

Consideration of the potential side-effects of antidepressants is important. When drugs are well tolerated the child's function and performance are not severely affected and as a result compliance is likely to be good. Most of the newer antidepressants are quite well tolerated, but a gradual introduction of medication also helps with this and similarly improves compliance.

As described in Chapter 3 the potential side-effects can be considered in terms of the effects on the different neurotransmitter systems (Table 16).

The extent to which the available antidepressants cause these effects is summarized in Table 17.

Table 16 Neurotransmitter effects and the adverse events they cause.

Neurotransmitter effect	Adverse effect	Clinical relevance
5-HT increase at 5-HT$_2$ receptors	Sleep disruption Sexual dysfuction Agitation	Try to avoid using drugs which have these effects when these symptoms are particularly problematic or have been caused by drugs before
5-HT increase at 5-HT$_3$ receptors	Nausea Diarrhoea Headache	Tolerance generally develops
NA increase	Tachycardia Sweating Insomnia	Best to avoid drugs which have these effects when these symptoms are particularly problematic or have been caused by drugs before
Decreased DA (because of interaction with 5-HT/NA or DA uptake)	Akathisia Other EPS	Avoid using drugs which have these effects in children with developmental problems or where there is evidence of minimal brain dysfunction
Cholinergic blockade	Blurred vision Constipation Dry mouth Drowsiness	Avoid using when these symptoms are important or there is a history of cardiac problems
α_1 receptor blockade	Postural hypotension Dizziness	Best to avoid when these symptoms are important
Histamine H$_1$ receptor blockade	Drowsiness Weight gain	Try to avoid using when these symptoms are important

Table 17 Effects of the different antidepressants on neurotransmitter systems.

Antidepressant	Increased NA symptoms	Increased 5-HT symptoms	5-HT$_2$ blocking effects	5-HT$_3$ blocking effects	Cholinergic blocking effects	α_1 blocking effects	Histamine blocking effects
TCA	++/+ Depending on TCA	++/− Depending on TCA	+/−	−	+++	+++	+++
SSRI	−	+++	−	−	−	−	−
Nefazodone	+	++	+++	−	−	−	−
Venlafaxine	++	+++	−	−	−	−	−
Moclobemide	++	++	−	−	−	−	−
Reboxetine	+++	−	−	−	−	−	−
Mirtazapine	+	+	+++	+++	−	−	+++

Formulation available

The availability of antidepressants in liquid formulation is particularly important for use in the young or in those who cannot tolerate tablets or express a preference for a liquid preparation.

Consideration of all these factors mean that it should be possible to make a sensible choice of which antidepressant to use. There is of course no precise recipe which can be followed for all cases but *Table 18* highlights some typical examples.

General guidelines

How long to treat?

Clinically a positive response from medication is frequently reported during the first 2 weeks, especially if the child or adolescent is going to benefit positively from the medication. An initial report of a slight lifting of mood is encouraging. In those who respond (typically 60–70 per cent of youngsters) medication should be continued at the dose that achieved this for at least a 6-month period *after* they report a marked improvement in their mood. This is a recommendation based on the current guidelines used in the treatment of adult depression.[47]

Discontinuing medication

Medication should never be stopped suddenly as the risk of withdrawal symptoms and the resurgence of sudden depression with vivid suicidal ideas have been reported. It is also sensible not to stop treatment at a time of particular stress, e.g. changing schools, and to always taper reductions in dose over a period of at least 2 weeks. Withdrawal problems typically occur 3–5 days after stopping medication abruptly and include dizziness, nausea and derealization. They have been reported most commonly with the abrupt discontinuation of paroxetine when they typically occur 3–5 days after stopping the drug. The likelihood of their

Table 18   Antidepressants for particular cases.

Presenting symptoms	Desired effects	Good choice
Moderate depression	Increased 5-HT or NA	SSRI/venlafaxine
Severe/retarded depression	Increased 5-HT and NA	Venlafaxine
Coexistent panic or OCD symptoms	Increased 5-HT	SSRI
Previous side-effects		
Insomnia	5-HT$_2$ blockade	Nefazodone/mirtazapine
Sexual problems	5-HT$_2$ blockade	
Agitation	5-HT$_2$ blockade	
Nausea	5-HT$_3$ blockade	Mirtazapine
GI disturbance	5-HT$_3$ blockade	

occurrence can however be limited by tapering the dose of antidepressant as described above.

Lack of response

About 30 per cent of children and adolescents fail to respond to the first-line antidepressant treatment. This lack of response may take the form of only partial resolution of symptoms or complete resistance to treatment. The youngster may well feel that they have failed in some way or be angry and upset that they will never get better. It is important to be systematic and to work through the treatment options in a consistent and logical way with a careful explanation at all stages. This gives everyone a sense of control and involves them in the whole treatment process. Difficult cases should always be treated seriously, the longer symptoms persist, the more intractable they become and the more resistant to treatment; time invested early should pay dividends later.

The plan for the treatment of those with resistant depression or those who have only partially responded is summarized in *Table 19*.

The first step is to review the whole case and treatment plan to elicit any unaddressed perpetuating factors, including non-compliance. The next step is to gradually titrate the antidepressant according to clinical response. In our view, if there is only limited or no improvement after 2–4 months at the full dose the antidepressant should be changed to one with effects on both 5-HT and NA, e.g. venlafaxine. The antidepressant should again be titrated up according to response and continued for at least 2 months. Care needs to be taken when switching from one antidepressant to another, as most are both metabolized by and interact with the P_{450} enzyme system (Chapter 3). This means that potentially toxic drug levels or a serotonergic syndrome can be produced with therapeutic doses.

Bearing this in mind, the speed at which you change antidepressants has to be driven by clinical need. If possible a time period of five times the half-life of the SSRI should be allowed for before starting on the new antidepressant. If however the clinical situation is more urgent, e.g. the young person is severely depressed, not eating or drinking, or is actively suicidal, then we would suggest halving the dose of the SSRI for 2 days

Table 19   Treating resistant depression.

Review the whole case, especially compliance, and consider a second opinion
Increase the dose of antidepressant
Consider   i) Changing the antidepressant
          ii) Augmentation strategies
            — Lithium
            — Thyroid hormones
            — Oestrogen therapy
          iii) ECT

and then stopping it. The venlafaxine can then be started at a dose of 37.5 mg once a day and titrated up according to response.

A second opinion at this stage is invaluable and should be sought.

Augmentation strategies

Augmentation strategies mean the addition of other medication to the antidepressant.

Of all the approaches there is most evidence for the efficacy of lithium augmentation which we would recommend as the first to use. Lithium needs to be introduced gradually and the dose titrated up with the aim of achieving lithium levels of 0.5–1.0 mmol/l. Routine blood investigations of renal and thyroid function should be performed before initiating lithium and regular blood tests performed until a stable level in this range is achieved. Some youngsters respond rapidly, i.e. within a few days, but a more typical pattern is for improvement to occur over a 2–3-week period. The lithium–antidepressant combination should therefore be continued for at least 2 months. Lithium augmentation can be used with all antidepressants, although the risk of a serotonin syndrome (Chapter 3) occurring with those antidepressants that target 5-HT means that this combination should be introduced cautiously.

If this fails, the next step is thyroid augmentation using tri-iodothyronine (T3) (or thyroxine (T4)), even in patients who are euthyroid.[48] As with lithium augmentation, dramatic rapid responses have been reported but a more usual pattern is for improvements to occur over several weeks. The combination should therefore be continued for at least 3 weeks. The T3 or T4 should be gradually titrated up whilst monitoring weight, pulse and ECG tracings when higher doses are used.

Augmentation with hormones such as oestrogen in the form of the contraceptive pill in females has been used successfully in some cases[49] (Masterson, personal communication).

ECT

This should only be considered by specialists working within tertiary centres and after at least one other second opinion has been sought. A recent review by Walters and Rey[50] outlines the current thinking regarding this form of treatment in children which should only be considered after all other avenues have failed.

Nonetheless, ECT therapeutic effect can be rapid in onset after even a single unilateral treatment and typically produces responses within a few days. The precise mechanism of action is unknown but it is thought to relate to the mobilization of neurotransmitters caused by the seizure.[51] In experimental animals, ECT downregulates β-receptors (analogous to antidepressants) but upregulates $5\text{-}HT_2$ receptors (opposite to antidepressants). Temporary memory loss and social stigma are the primary problems with ECT.

Maintenance therapy

As mentioned earlier, many patients have chronic and recurrent mood disorders which require maintenance therapy. Good clinical practice is to select the same antidepressant that improved the child's condition and to use it at the same dose (previous older recommendations had been to halve the dose). Deciding who will need maintenance therapy is a matter of clinical judgement. The risks and benefits of treatment need to be carefully weighed against the risks associated with the illness. Account needs to be taken of the child's clinical presentation and their suicide risk when unwell, the presence of any salient aetiological or perpetuating factors, the effects of discontinuation of medication previously and their family psychiatric history. In some cases it is clear that stopping medication would very likely result in a relapse which may well have serious and possibly life-threatening consequences.

Treating bipolar disorder

Mood stabilizers

The mood stablizers (lithium, carbamazepine, sodium valproate) have shown proven efficacy in the treatment of children with manic or hypomanic symptoms. They have also been proven as maintenance treatments for bipolar disorder. Their use as augmentation medications for cases of resistant depression is based on the adult literature.

Lithium

Lithium remains the mainstay of maintenance treatment for bipolar disorders.

Before starting treatment, it is important to assess baseline renal and thyroid functions.

Lithium carbonate is the form most often used and should be started at a low dose, e.g. 200 mg (5.4 mmol Li^+) mané after food for the first 3 days increased to 200 mg twice-daily (for an adolescent over 45 kg). A twelve hour post-dose blood sample should be taken after 4–7 days and the dosage altered accordingly to obtain an optimal level. The aim is to achieve a therapeutic plasma level of lithium of between 0.5 and 1.0 mmol/l. Weekly tests continue until a steady level has been achieved and then testing can be performed every 3 months. Low dose and twice-daily dosing reduce the likelihood of side-effects but, once stable, single daily administration can be used to ease administration and improve compliance. Side-effects include GI disturbances, fine tremor, and weight gain. Advice, including a lithium treatment card, should be dispensed to warn of lithium toxicity, especially during intercurrent infections with diarrhoea and vomiting.

Carbamazepine

Carbamazepine has a clinical place in the treatment of bipolar disorders and can be considered when lithium does not work or in cases of rapid cycling. It can be prescribed initially at doses of 100 mg twice-daily after food and increased after 7 days to 200 mg twice-daily if necessary. By introducing the medication more slowly, side-effects are again minimized. A blood level will direct the clinician on how best to titrate the dose to obtain the optimum therapeutic level between 20 and 50 μmol/l.

Common side-effects include nausea, vomiting, dizziness and drowsiness or ataxia. Particular note should be taken of any persistent sore throat whilst on medication and a FBC taken to exclude blood dyscrasia.

Sodium valproate

Sodium valproate can also be used as a maintenance treatment for bipolar disorders and again should be considered when lithium fails to produce a response. It can be prescribed at doses of 100–200 mg at night, increasing up to 20 mg/kg, usually in divided doses. Monitoring blood levels can be useful to aid titration and check compliance.

Antipsychotics

Currently available antipsychotics do have a role in the treatment of bipolar disorders in children and adolescents, although the data from well-controlled, randomized studies are limited.

Sulpiride, risperidone and olanzapine have shown promising results in the treatment of acute mania.[52] Hepatotoxicity has been reported with risperidone, although this was found to be reversible on withdrawal of the drug.[53]

5
Anxiety disorders

Anxiety disorders can be as complex as mood disorders and are likewise most appropriately treated within the context of a Child and Adolescent Mental Health Service (CAMHS) using the skills of the multidisciplinary team.

The classification of anxiety has changed considerably since 1980, when the concept of these disorders occurring in children was first introduced into DSM III. Before this, anxiety symptoms had been included in a behavioural disorder category in a non-specific way. The DSM III schedule provided three diagnostic anxiety groups: separation anxiety disorder, avoidant anxiety disorder and overanxious disorder. It also recognized that other anxiety disorders occurring in adults, including obsessive-compulsive disorder (OCD), panic disorder, phobias, and post-traumatic stress disorder (PTSD), could begin in childhood. When DSM IV was introduced in 1994, the only distinct childhood anxiety disorder remaining was separation anxiety disorder, as the other two groups (avoidant anxiety disorder and overanxious disorder) became broadly incorporated into the diagnoses of social phobia and generalized anxiety disorder. These differences between DSM III and DSM IV are summarized in *Table 20*.

Perhaps one of the most important aspects of the DSM evolution of anxiety disorders in children has been its emphasis on the continuity of disorders between childhood and adulthood. Epidemiological research on anxiety disorder classification in adolescence reveals that there are

Table 20   Differences between DSM III and DSM IV.

DSM III	DSM IV
Separation anxiety disorder	Separation anxiety disorder
Avoidant anxiety disorder	Social phobia
Overanxious anxiety disorder	Generalized anxiety disorder

Table 21   Anxiety disorders and ages of onset (according to DSM IV).

Disorder	Age of onset
Panic disorder	May begin in childhood; peak onset late adolescence to early 20s
Social anxiety disorder	Median age of onset 13 years
Obsessive-compulsive disorder	Usual onset males 6–15 years, females 20–29 years
Post-traumatic stress disorder	Any age
Generalized anxiety disorder	Many begin in childhood/ adolescence
Acute stress disorder	Any age
Specific phobia	Peak onset in childhood (age 5 years)

clear links with adult anxiety and mood disorders. Although most psychiatric conditions occurring in early childhood have resolved by adulthood, it is frequently found that adult anxiety or mood disorders are preceded by a similar condition in adolescence. It is important that the child psychiatrist be aware of the classification of adult anxiety disorders if a true longitudinal clinical perspective is to be realized. *Table 21* lists the main disorders in the DSM IV classification.

The delineation of the various anxiety disorders has been accompanied by a wealth of studies that have investigated the biological underpinning of these similar but separate disorders. We cannot do justice here to the many established psychological theories regarding the aetiology of such disorders which range from the psychodynamic to cognitive behaviour. For the purpose of this discussion we will only focus on the biological and pharmacological perspectives. Many of the published studies emphasize subtle differences in neurotransmitter function among the disorders that mirror discrete but important clinical differences. This has several implications, ensures that the diagnosis is correct, and that, if drug treatment is used, it is based on sound and developing theoretical knowledge.

Obsessive-compulsive disorder

Although OCD is the best studied anxiety disorder in childhood, it still remains both under-diagnosed and under-treated despite the fact that it is very amenable to treatment. Frequently, there is a long delay between the onset of symptoms and the young person seeking help. In a large study of OCD involving more than 700 patients, a mean treatment gap of 17 years was found between symptom onset (at age 14–15 years) and correct diagnosis.[54]

OCD is defined in both ICD-10 and DSM-IV as repetitive, intrusive thoughts and/or rituals that are unwanted and which interfere significantly with functions or cause marked distress. Recognition that the obsessions or compulsions are unreasonable, and the severity and disabling nature of the disorder helps to differentiate the condition from normal childhood development. It should also be emphasized that children do not often request help; it is usually parents who identify the associated behavioural symptoms whatever the presentation. Early diagnosis is essential in order to prevent secondary complications, such as impaired peer and family relationships or collusion and disrupted education.

The common obsessive thoughts reported are similar to those found in adults with OCD which include the fear of contamination and the fear of danger to oneself or another person *(Table 22)*. The most common compulsions are also similar to those seen in adults, e.g. excessive washing and repetitive rituals such as checking and touching.

Prevalence

The prevalence rate for OCD in adolescents is of the order of 1 per cent, with a lifetime prevalence of 1.9 per cent. It is important to note that approximately a third to half of adults with the disorder present with symptoms before the age of 15. There are some important gender differences. Males appear to predominate in pre-pubertal cases, but the sex ratio levels out in adolescence. Males tend to present earlier and have more severe symptoms at presentation. Early-onset OCD appears to be more highly familial and is associated with a distinct pattern of comorbid psychopathology.

Comorbidity

A longitudinal prospective follow-up study of 25 children and adolescents with OCD[55] revealed high comorbidity at 2–7-year follow-up. Common comorbid disorders included tic disorder, mood disorders, overanxious disorder and oppositional disorder *(Table 23)*.

Aetiology of OCD

Neurochemical
Several lines of evidence point to the involvement of the serotonergic system in OCD. Much of this evidence comes from empirical studies which show that the only effective psychopharmacological treatments for OCD are with drugs that act on the serotonergic system.

A now classic study in adults[56] investigated the tricyclic antidepressant clomipramine (serotonergic) versus desipramine (noradrenergic) in a double-blind crossover trial. Clomipramine was significantly superior to desipramine, and 64 per cent of patients who received clomipramine as their first active drug showed evidence of relapse when switched over to desipramine *(Figure 25)*.

Table 22   Major presenting obsessive compulsions and thoughts in 70 children and adolescents with severe OCD.

Compulsions		Thoughts	
Handwashing, showering or grooming	85%	Concern with dirt/germs	40%
Repeating	51%	Something terrible happening	24%
Checking	46%	Symmetry, order	17%
Removing contact with contaminants	23%	Scrupulousness	13%
Touching	20%	Concern with bodily secretions	8%
Counting	18%		

Results of NIMH study of 70 children and adolescents with severe OCD.[57]

Table 23 Figures of comorbidity of 25 children and adolescents on re-evaluation at 2–7-year follow-up.[55]

Disorder	Percentage
Tic disorder	59
Major depression	56
Overanxious disorder	54
Oppositional disorder	30

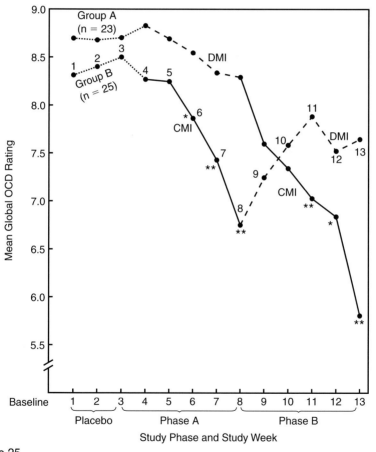

Figure 25

Weekly scores on the National Institute of Mental Health global obsessive-compulsive disorder (OCD) rating scale during placebo, desipramine hydrochloride (DMI), and clomipramine hydrochloride (CMI) treatment periods. Single asterisk indicates $P < 0.05$ by Bonferroni t statistic; double asterisk, $P < 0.01$ by Bonferroni t statistic.[56]

Furthermore, a double-blind crossover study of clomipramine versus placebo[58] in 19 children with severe OCD showed significant improvement of obsessive symptoms with clomipramine. Symptom improvement was directly correlated with pre-treatment platelet serotonin concentration, which decreased following treatment with clomipramine.

Further evidence for serotonergic abnormalities includes the finding that serotonin transporter protein (measured peripherally in platelets) is significantly reduced in children and adolescents with OCD compared with controls.[59]

Neuroanatomical

A number of neuropsychiatric conditions can present with obsessive-compulsive behaviour. This aids our understanding of the possible underlying specific neuropathological abnormalities and implicates the basal ganglia in particular.

Paediatric autoimmune neuropsychiatric disorders (PANDAS), including Sydenham's chorea, are of particular interest in our understanding of child and adolescent OCD. Sydenham's chorea is associated with rheumatic fever and is thought to result from cross-reaction of autoimmune antibodies to β-haemolytic *Streptococcus* with caudate neurones in the basal ganglia. In two retrospective studies of patients with Sydenham's chorea, high numbers of patients with obsessive symptomatology were found, despite no premorbid history of obsessions. Obsessive symptoms were concomitant with chorea and remitted before cessation of the choreiform movements. Subjects did not go on to develop further obsessive behaviour, suggesting a discrete episode related to the presence of antineuronal antibodies.[60,61] Another recent study[62] provides further support for this hypothesis. Children with severe infection-triggered exacerbations of OCD or tic disorders had reduced severity of neuropsychiatric symptoms following treatment with either plasma exchange or intravenous immunoglobulin (IVIG) compared with placebo. Global change scores at 1 month follow-up were improved by 48 per cent and 41 per cent in the plasma exchange and IVIG groups, respectively, compared with no change in the placebo group. A very recent study has however cast some doubt over the association with antistreptococcal antibodies suggesting that these are also found in ADHD and the presence of this condition may have compounded the previous findings.[63]

Neuroimaging data in adults tells us something about OCD pathology. Magnetic resonance imaging (MRI) of subjects with early-onset OCD reveals structural caudate nucleus abnormalities, but functional scanning gives more useful information on the pathophysiology of the disorder. Metabolic scanning studies have suggested hypermetabolism in the orbitofrontal cortex, anterior cingulate gyrus, caudate nuclei and thalamus in adults with OCD. Studies have also looked at cerebral bloodflow following treatment response and largely reported a decrease in caudate and orbitofrontal hypermetabolism. A classic study in this field[64] also showed abnormalities in metabolism in the caudate nuclei, orbitofrontal cortex and thalamus in adult OCD patients which were reduced following successful treatment with both drug and behavioural therapy.

Two very recent MRI studies in children aged 8–17 years with OCD have confirmed some but not all of the adult findings and reported significantly greater thalamic volumes in those with OCD compared with controls.[65,66] Interestingly some of these young people were followed up after treatment with either an SSRI, paroxetine[65] or CBT.[66] Those who had responded to treatment with paroxetine were found to have a decrease in thalamic volume. The same changes were not, however, found in those who responded to treatment with CBT with no difference in thalamic volume being found before or after treatment with CBT.

One MRI study of children with OCD or tics associated with a streptococcal injection has reported an enlargement of the basal ganglia (but not the thalamus) in this distinct subgroup of subjects with OCD.[67] These findings are consistent with the hypothesis of an autoimmune response to streptococcal injection (described above).

Genetic factors

Family genetic studies have repeatedly shown that OCD is familial and that sub-threshold OCD (symptoms not causing marked distress or dysfunction) also has familial inheritance. However, it is important to recognize that not all cases of OCD follow this pattern; and even in studies that have shown high rates of OCD in first-degree relatives, the majority of probands have no affected first-degree relatives.[68]

There has only been one twin study published. This looked at 15 monozygotic (MZ) and 15 dizygotic (DZ) twin pairs, and showed concordance rates for treated OCD of 33 per cent and 7 per cent, respectively. These figures increased if the phenotype was broadened to include OCD symptoms, regardless of the need for treatment.[57]

Assessment

A thorough assessment is again the key to making a clear diagnosis. The nature of the presenting problems needs to be carefully identified.

It is important when assessing young people to be aware that they can perceive obsessive symptoms as extremely embarrassing. It is common, therefore, for children to practise their obsessive rituals secretly which means that it is very helpful to speak to parents, teachers, etc. who can provide good collateral information on a child's level of functioning and distress. It is also important to elicit whether family members are involved or have inadvertently colluded with the child or adolescent's symptoms, as this has important implications for treatment.

Assessment of obsessive-compulsive symptoms should ideally include the use of a symptom severity rating scales such as the modified Child Yale Brown Obsessive Compulsive scale (CY-BOCS). The main difference between the childhood and adult scales is that the children's scale uses information from both child and parent. It has good reliability for obsessions and acceptable reliability for compulsions and is regarded as the best rating scale for both clinical and research purposes. It can be completed at the initial assessment to give a baseline, and during and after treatment to monitor progress and outcome respectively.

It is also important to perform a physical examination before treatment, including recording a measure of height, weight and blood pressure (sitting and standing), as well as baseline blood investigations, such as tests for full blood count (FBC), erythrocyte sedimentation rate (ESR), C reactive protein (CRP), urea and electrolytes (U&Es), antistreptolysin (ASO titres), and thyroid function tests (TFTs). Although rarely abnormal they may rule out comorbid disorders and act as a baseline.

Having made the diagnosis, the young person and family need to be informed about the condition and the factors that play a part in its aetiology and maintenance. Information regarding the natural history and course of the disorder, the risks and benefits associated with the various treatment options and the expected length of treatment should also be discussed.

Treatment

Psychological treatment
Although psychopharmacological treatments are our focus here and are an essential aspect of treatment, they should be considered in conjunction with psychological treatments, particularly behavioural therapy (which includes exposure and response prevention) and family intervention therapy. Psychoeducation and externalizing techniques can also be helpful, e.g. using a nickname for the obsessive symptoms.

Psychopharmacological treatments
Drugs which act on the serotonergic system are effective in the treatment of OCD.

TCAs
Clomipramine is the most serotonergic of the tricyclics and the most studied tricyclic in the treatment of OCD in adults and children. There have been two placebo-controlled clinical trials of clomipramine in the treatment of OCD in children and adolescents and one trial of clomipramine versus desipramine that demonstrate good efficacy.

A 10-week double-blind crossover trial of clomipramine versus placebo[58] in 12 children with severe OCD found significant improvement for clomipramine over placebo on both observed and self-reported symptoms at 3 and 5 weeks, irrespective of baseline depressive symptoms. A further placebo-controlled study[69] showed a mean reduction on CY-BOCS rating of 37 per cent in the clomipramine group (75–200 mg/day) compared with 8 per cent in the placebo group in an 8-week multicentre study of 60 children and adolescents with OCD. The double blind crossover trial of clomipramine vs desipramine cited earlier[56] also demonstrated a significant benefit for those taking clomipramine.

High peak plasma levels of clomipramine are associated with an increased incidence of side-effects. It is therefore important to introduce the medication slowly, to help minimize the occurrence of these. A typical dose for a child is between 75 and 150 mg/day, with the usual dose for an adolescent ranging from 100–250 mg/day.

Common side-effects of clomipramine are listed in *Table 24*. Perhaps of most concern are the potential cardiotoxic side-effects and reports of sudden death in patients on tricyclics, although to date no causal relationship has been established and nor have any sudden deaths been reported in children prescribed clomipramine. It is, however, important to conduct a baseline electrocardiogram (ECG) before commencing treatment, together with a measurement of baseline heart rate and blood pressure (and repeating this 3–4 days after each dose increment). The value of maintenance ECG monitoring at 4–6-monthly intervals has not been established but is recommended by some. It is also important to avoid rapid withdrawal of the drug as this can cause a recognized withdrawal syndrome and occasionally precipitate seizures.

SSRIs

Although clomipramine is the best studied drug treatment in childhood OCD, the newer selective serotonin reuptake inhibitors (SSRIs) are showing promising results and less cardio and neurotoxic effects.

Table 24   Common side-effects of clomipramine.

Dry mouth
Blurred vision
Postural hypotension
Constipation
Elevated resting heart rate
Weight gain
Sweating
Delayed micturition
Headache
Tremor
Drowsiness

Fluvoxamine is licensed in the USA for the treatment of OCD in both adults and children (aged 8–17 years). Its efficacy has been demonstrated in a double-blind, placebo-controlled multicentre study of 120 children and adolescents, with group differences being noticed after just 1 week.[68] Although the most dramatic improvement was in the first 3 weeks, this response continued throughout the 10-week study. In an earlier, open-label study[40] of 20 adolescent inpatients with OCD, subjects showed a significant response to fluvoxamine, including those with comorbid Tourette's syndrome or schizophrenia (for which they also received haloperidol).

Children and adolescents in a placebo-controlled trial of fluoxetine (20 mg/day) showed symptomatic improvement (44 per cent) compared with placebo (27 per cent), although the sample size was small and the fixed dosage may have been too high for this population.[70] Improvement of both obsessions and compulsions in the seven subjects receiving fluoxetine was evident after 4 weeks of treatment. Side-effects reported included insomnia (55 per cent), motor activation (27 per cent), and nausea (27 per cent) *(Table 25)*. Interestingly, fluoxetine exacerbated motor tics in two children with these at baseline.

The largest psychopharmacological study in this age group has been with sertraline. This was a multicentre study of 107 children (aged 6–12 years) and 80 adolescents (aged 13–17 years) and compared the efficacy of sertraline (maximum dose 200 mg/day) with placebo for 12 weeks. The results reported that the sertraline treated group showed significantly greater improvement than placebo on all the rating scales used. At the end of the 12 week study 42 per cent of those receiving sertraline compared with 26 per cent of those on placebo were very much or much improved. The side effects reported by those on sertraline were similar to those on other SSRIs, i.e. insomnia, nausea and agitations.[71]

A large multicentre trial with paroxetine is currently underway in the USA.

More recent, open-label studies have examined the efficacy of citalopram, the most selective of the available SSRIs. Results are also promis-

Table 25   Common side-effects of SSRIs.

Symptom	Receptor responsible
Insomnia	$5\text{-}HT_2$
Motor activation	$5\text{-}HT_2$
Sexual dysfunction	$5\text{-}HT_2$
Diarrhoea	$5\text{-}HT_3$
Nausea	$5\text{-}HT_3$
Headache	$5\text{-}HT_3$

ing, and it appears to be particularly well tolerated in children and adolescents with OCD. Randomized, double-blind, placebo-controlled trials are now required to establish efficacy.[72]

Generally, the SSRIs are well tolerated in children and adolescents, especially if low doses are used initially and dose titration is gradual. As SSRIs do not block other receptors, unlike the TCAs, they are generally better tolerated and, importantly, safer. Side-effects occur because 5-HT acts on a number of different receptors. Increased throughput at the 5-HT_2 receptor causes insomnia, motor activation and sexual dysfunction; 5-HT_3 stimulation results in gastrointestinal (GI) disturbances, including nausea, abdominal discomfort, diarrhoea and vomiting (although rare and self-limiting) and headaches (Table 25). Behavioural activation and agitation is more problematic in children than adults, although this appears to be dose-dependent and transient.[68]

General guidelines

The choice of drug treatment is between the TCA, clomipramine and one of the SSRIs. Although clomipramine has been the most extensively studied, because of its side effects, the first choice is usually a SSRI. In general it is best to start with a low dose and to increase this very gradually until symptom relief is sustained or side-effects intervene (Table 26).

The studies detailed above suggest that high doses of all antidepressant are usually required for benefit. This is similar to findings from the adult literature, which also recommend a long duration of treatment, often up to a year.

Treatment of OCD with comorbid Tourette's syndrome and other tic disorders
The anti-obsessive effects of the SSRIs is less pronounced in children or adolescents with comorbid tic disorders. There have been reports of exacerbation of pre-existing tic disorders with the use of SSRIs for comorbid OCD. In these cases addition of a neuroleptic, e.g. haloperidol or an atypical antipsychotic is often effective in reducing tics although one author reported that risperidone could exacerabate OCD symptoms in some adolescents.[73]

Treatment of OCD with comorbid depression
Where OCD occurs with comorbid depression, the first-line treatment should be an SSRI as studies suggest that this is an effective treatment for both depression and OCD. However, the dose may need to be titrated cautiously in children and adolescents to minimize side-effects.

Table 26 Summary of double blind psychopharmacological studies of OCD in children and adolescents. Adapted from MF Flament InsermmU302, Hopital La Salpetriere, Paris, France.

Reference	Drug	Dose	Number	Duration
Flament et al[58]	Clomipramine	100–200 mg	19	10 weeks
Leonard et al[56]	Clomipramine	Mean = 150 mg	47	5 weeks
	Cross over with desipramine	Mean = 153 mg		5 weeks
DeVeaugh-Geiss et al[69]	Clomipramine	75–200 mg	60	8 weeks
Riddle et al[70]	Fluoxetine	20 mg	14	8 weeks + 12 weeks
March et al[71]	Sertraline	200 mg	187	12 weeks
Riddle et al[68]	Fluvoxamine	50–200 mg	120	10 weeks

Social anxiety disorder

Social anxiety disorder (also called social phobia) is defined as a persistent fear of situations in which the person is exposed to public scrutiny. They fear they may act in a way that will be humiliating or embarrassing. Exposure to these social situations almost invariably triggers an immediate anxiety response that sometimes fulfils the criteria for a full-blown panic attack. The disorder may be either circumscribed (e.g. a particular performance anxiety) or be much more generalized (occurring in a range of social situations).

The onset of social anxiety disorder is often in adolescence yet it often presents much later with the development of a comorbid disorder, such as substance abuse or major depression. Adult studies suggest that the frequent self medication with alcohol and subsequent alcohol dependence could be prevented. Approximately 25 per cent of adults presenting with social anxiety disorder have a comorbid diagnosis of alcohol dependency.[74] The ready availability and social acceptability of alcohol, together with its acute anxiolytic effect, mean that people frequently self-medicate in order to reduce anxiety. Increased tolerance and mild dependency following a gradual increase in the amount of alcohol consumed in order to combat the social phobia or symptoms of anxiety following withdrawal can lead to full-blown alcohol dependency usually presenting in the 3rd or 4th decade (Figure 20). Social anxiety disorder is probably the commonest treatable cause of alcohol dependency in young men.

Prevalence

The current prevalence figures for social anxiety disorder are between 1% and 7% in children and adolescents, with a mean age of onset between 11–15 years. Long-term studies suggest that the clinical course is chronic, lasting into adulthood.

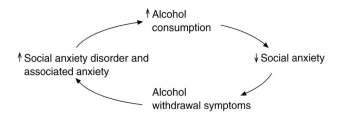

Figure 26
Self medication with alcohol and social anxiety.

Comorbidity

In addition to alcohol abuse, social anxiety disorder also appears to have high comorbidity with substance misuse (e.g. stimulants) and with other disorders of anxiety, mood and personality.

Aetiology

Much of our understanding of the psychobiology of social anxiety disorder (albeit limited) comes from adult studies.[75]

Neurochemical

The neurotransmitters implicated in social anxiety disorder include noradrenaline (NA), serotonin (5-HT), and dopamine (DA).[76]

The evidence for NA involvement is mixed. Those with specific social phobias (but not generalized) have a greater increase in heart rate in response to the behavioural challenge of public speaking. There is also some evidence of altered autonomic reactivity, with increased blood pressure responsivity to the valsalva manoeuvre and a reduction in the normal blood pressure drop that occurs on standing.

The evidence for 5-HT dysfunction is more substantial. Again, much of this comes from empirical treatment studies which show that drugs with effects on 5-HT (MAOIs, RIMAs and SSRIs) are all effective. Neuroendocrine studies in adults which were challenged with the 5-HT partial agonist m-CPP and the 5-HT-releasing agent fenfluramine reported an increase in cortisol responses, which suggests postsynaptic serotonergic hypersensitivity.[77]

Social anxiety disorder is the only one of the anxiety disorders in which there is clear evidence of dopaminergic dysfunction. One of the best pieces of research evidence comes from an imaging study showing decreased dopamine reuptake site density in the striatum of adults with social anxiety disorder compared with controls.[78] This may explain why those who misuse stimulant drugs (such as amphetamine) report a reduction of social anxiety because these drugs increase dopamine levels.

Assessment

Again, the cornerstone of treatment is a thorough assessment. The symptoms of social anxiety disorder in children and adolescents appear consistent with those seen in adulthood. Children and adolescents with social anxiety disorder have higher trait anxiety than the normal population and report subjective symptoms of anxiety when engaged in socially exposing activities, such as reading aloud or performing in front of their classmates. Such activities will frequently lead to emotional distress, the development of somatic symptoms, and subsequent behavioural avoidance. Selective mutism, the failure to talk in specific social situations (e.g. the classroom) while talking in other places, is regarded by some as part of the socially phobic presentation in children. Following a study conducted in 30 children with selective mutism 97 per cent were shown to fulfil a diagnosis of social phobia it has been suggested that selective mutism is in fact a symptom of social anxiety rather than a distinct diagnostic syndrome.[79]

The difficulty in diagnosing social anxiety disorder in children and adolescents is likely to be due to its under-recognition by both children/parents and professionals, compounded by the lack of adequate rating scales. There are no specific rating scales for social phobia in children and adolescents so clinicians have to resort to general anxiety scales, (Spank Children's Anxiety self-rating scale or Hamilton Anxiety Rating Scale (HARS)), and behavioural scales such as the Children's Behavioural Check List (CBCL). The adult scales which rate specific social phobic symptoms may also be useful (Liebowitz, SPIN) but they need some modification for use in this age group. It is also important to acquire collateral histories from the parents or main carers to provide a comprehensive picture. It is interesting to note that children of socially phobic parents have a greatly increased risk of developing a psychiatric disorder, especially an anxiety disorder, which emphasizes the importance of obtaining a full family psychiatric history.

On a more practical level, it can be useful to build up a series of age-appropriate questions to help to establish a diagnosis in a child with social anxiety disorder. Close questioning about the child's anxiety in the classroom when placed under the spotlight may be revealing especially if the child reports severe symptoms of anxiety and distress. They are likely to place themselves in the least conspicuous place in the class and avoid situations that would expose them to their classmates. It is helpful to ask about blushing, as this can strengthen the diagnosis and can differentiate the diagnosis of social anxiety disorder from panic disorder, when the child or adolescent typically appears pale in colour.

Useful interview questions to ask are as follows:

- Ask where the child sits in the classroom.
- Ask if the child ever volunteers to do something in class in front of others. Ask what happens if the teacher asks the child to read aloud or write in front of others.
- Ask whether the child tends to blush in anxiety-provoking situations.

Psycho-education for the staff in schools is very important to prevent the child developing secondary avoidance behaviour, including school refusal. It is essential to consider social anxiety disorder when seeing any child who is presenting with school refusal.

Treatment

Unfortunately there are very few published data on the efficacy of treatments for children and adolescents with social anxiety disorder which may be partially related to the relatively short time that social anxiety disorder has been accepted as a diagnosis in this age group. Many of the data are, therefore, extrapolated from adult studies.

Psychological treatments

The rationale for psychological treatments in this population partially relies on evaluation of existing literature examining behavioural exposure, cognitive restructuring, and social skills training for shy children and adolescents. This, along with extrapolation of findings from adult studies, suggests a place for cognitive-behavioural therapy.

Psychopharmacological treatments

If clinical improvement is still limited after the implementation of psychological techniques, it is worth considering medication, although the experimental nature of the treatment needs to be explained to the family. Although it is difficult to conclusively recommend drug treatment for children and adolescents with social anxiety disorder, several treatment options are available.

These include a RIMA (reversible monoamine oxidase inhibitor), e.g. moclobemide, an SSRI, or a high-potency benzodiazepine (although concerns remain about the dependence potential as well as the more frequent reports of drowsiness and oppositional behaviour compared to those described in adults). TCAs are not effective.

Moclobemide

Moclobemide is the only RIMA available in the UK and is licensed for the treatment of this disorder in adults. However there have been no studies conducted on children and adolescents on the effectiveness of moclobemide and social anxiety disorder. Although traditional MAOIs are an option in adults they should not be used in children because of the well-established and potentially dangerous 'cheese reaction' and the higher risk of orthostatic hypotension.

SSRIs

SSRIs also appear to be effective and promising results from adult studies have been reported. An open-label study of fluoxetine in 21 children with separation anxiety disorder, social anxiety disorder or overanxious disorder showed that 81 per cent had a marked to moderate improvement after 12 weeks.[80] An open-label study of fluoxetine conducted on 21 children with selective mutism (10–60 mg/day) showed that 76 per cent improved, with diminished anxiety and increased ability to speak publicly.[81]

β-*Blockers*

β-Blockers are effective in reducing autonomic-mediated symptoms, such as tremor and palpitations, but have little effect on subjective symptoms of anxiety. They play a useful role in circumscribed, performance-related social anxiety disorder, e.g. for musicians, but are of limited value for the group with symptoms of more generalized social anxiety. They can also precipitate asthmatic attacks in sensitive subjects and are associated with other side-effects.

Panic disorder

Panic disorder is one of the most severe presentations of anxiety and in adults is associated with high levels of morbidity and increased mortality. It is defined in DSM IV as: recurrent, unexpected panic attacks associated with a 1-month history of persistent apprehension about a further attack; worry about the implications of a further attack; or significant change in behaviour related to an attack. Although it usually begins in early adulthood, it is frequently associated with antecedent childhood distress such as excessive fearfulness and separation anxiety. The symptoms of a panic attack are listed in *Table 27*.

Prevalence

Despite the fact that the typical age of onset of panic disorder is in the late teens or early 20's it has recently been shown that panic disorder can emerge in childhood and early adolescence. Prevalence rates of 5.4 per cent have been noted in a community sample of 13–18 year olds. The disorder has significant clinical implications and if left untreated follows a chronic, disabling course.

Table 27   Symptoms of a panic attack.

Palpitations or tachycardia
Sweating
Trembling or shaking
Sensations of shortness of breath or smothering
Feelings of choking
Chest pain or discomfort
Nausea or abdominal distress
Feeling dizzy, light-headed, or faint
Derealization/depersonalization
Fear of losing control or going crazy
Fear of dying
Paraesathesias

Comorbidity

Although there is limited research and literature available on juvenile panic disorder there are similarities with the adult form of the disorder in particular a high comorbid incidence of agoraphobia or other anxiety and mood disorders.

Aetiology

Neurochemical

The biological basis for panic disorder was first hypothesized following the results of challenge studies with lactate which reliably precipitated panic attack symptoms in those with a panic disorder but not normal controls.[82] Since then, a variety of other panic-inducing agents have been identified which produce similar results, carbon dioxide (CO_2), cholecystokinin (CCK), the benzodiazepine antagonist, flumazenil, and the α_2 antagonist, yohimbine. These findings suggest that those with panic disorder have some biological susceptibility to panic attacks, although the precise nature of the abnormalities involved have yet to be determined.

Research in adults suggest that several neurotransmitters are implicated, including NA, 5-HT and GABA. There is also evidence that respiratory and cardiovascular reactivity is abnormal.

Noradrenergic abnormalities are suggested by results from challenge studies with α_2-antagonists and agonists. The α_2-antagonist yohimbine, which increases the level of NA in the synapse, produces panic symptoms in those with panic disorder but not in healthy volunteers. This suggests those with panic disorder have an increased NA sensitivity. Studies with the α_2-agonist clonidine have shown blunted growth hormone responses suggesting reduced postsynaptic receptor sensitivity which may be a reflection of receptor down-regulation as a consequence of increased NA in the synapse. At the present time, no single explanation clearly delineates the role of NA in panic disorder. It is most likely to have a role in the symptoms of heightened arousal, anticipatory fear and hypervigilance.

The role of 5-HT in panic is also not clearly determined (reviewed in Bell and Nutt[83]). 5-HT abnormalities are suggested empirically by the clinical efficacy of serotonergic drugs, e.g. SSRIs. Preclinical studies suggest that receptors may be hypersensitive (as shown by the effects of neuroendocrine challenges with, for example, m-CPP and fenfluramine), but most explanations point to the fact that different brain regions and receptors are involved in different ways.

GABA is the most common neurotransmitter in the brain. It acts on the GABA-A benzodiazepine receptor (GBzR), which also has binding sites for barbiturates, alcohol and benzodiazepines. It is the main inhibitory receptor system in the brain, and agonists at the receptor cause a reduction in anxiety, an increase in seizure threshold, and sedation (see Chapter 3). There is evidence which suggests that the sensitivity of the GABA-A benzodiazepine receptor is reduced in panic disorder.[84] A recent positron emission tomography (PET) study has also shown a decrease in GBzR binding in adult patients with panic disorder[85] which adds to earlier work suggesting functional abnormality in this system.

Assessment

The very physical nature of the symptoms of panic attacks means that they are frequently misdiagnosed with several clinicians being consulted before the diagnosis is made. Some children somatize and are less able to express physical sensations, which may further complicate the diagnostic process. Nonetheless the exclusion of other physical disorders is a prerequisite.

Adolescents presenting with the disorder are often mistakenly diagnosed as having a physical disorder such as asthma and in some cases inappropriately treated. In one study[86] researchers found that 36 per cent of the 28 adolescents with panic disorder presented with other symptoms obscuring the presence of panic attacks. Interestingly a third of the 21 females in the study presented with refusal to eat and nausea.

Diagnosis can be hampered further by the child's developmental level and associated limitations in cognitive understanding of complex symptoms such as depersonalization. Children are more prone to give non-catastrophic interpretations of a panic attack, unlike their adolescent and adult counterparts. It also seems that panic attacks in children are less likely to occur 'out of the blue'.[87] A diagnosis should, therefore, be entertained in children with a recent history of anxiety symptoms associated with avoidant behaviours, such as school refusal.

When assessing a child or adolescent, it is useful to consider the three cardinal features of panic disorder: panic attacks, anticipatory anxiety, and phobic avoidance. The use of a panic diary can be helpful in obtaining a baseline, as well as monitoring the effects of treatment. The child and carers can be helped to identify examples of phobic avoidance, once this feature has been explained. Helpful questions include asking where the child chooses to sit in class, as those with a disorder will often prefer a seat nearest to the door in order to ensure a quick exit should a panic attack occur.

Interview questions for assessment of juvenile panic disorder are as follows:

- Ask for a description of the 'panic attacks'.
- Ask about behavioural avoidance, e.g. preferred place in the classroom.
- Assess levels of anticipatory anxiety by using visual analogue scales.

Treatment

Psychological

There are no published data on psychological treatments for juvenile panic disorder although preliminary evidence suggests that techniques used in adults may be useful. Cognitive-behavioural therapy (CBT) is the most established modality of treatment.

Psychopharmacological treatments

Until evaluative, controlled, clinical trials have been conducted on the paediatric population for anxiety disorders, clinicians must extrapolate from the results of the existing research and literature in the adult population. The options include TCAs, SSRIs and benzodiazepines.

TCAs

Imipramine and clomipramine appear to be efficacious in the treatment of panic disorder and for a long time were the mainstays of treatment. As mentioned in Chapter 3 *(Figure 16)* these are the most serotonergic of the TCAs. The major problem with these drugs are their side-effects, which lead to high drop-out rates in adult controlled trials. This is also likely to be an important factor in children and adolescents. An initial exacerbation of symptoms at the start of treatment often occurs. Treatment should therefore be initiated with a low starting dose and titrated slowly.

SSRIs

Several randomized, controlled trials have demonstrated the efficacy of SSRIs in adult patients with panic disorder; and both paroxetine and citalopram are now licensed for this. Although the efficacy of SSRIs cannot be assumed in the paediatric population, they are generally perceived as being preferable to tricyclics. They are better tolerated, have fewer cardiovascular complications, and are safer following overdose. Since there is often an exacerbation of symptoms when treatment is initiated it is best to start at a low dose and increase after 1–2 weeks. It is important to explain that there may be an exacerbation of symptoms over the first few days and a high-potency benzodiazepine such as clonazepam can be prescribed for 1–2 weeks (e.g. 0.5 mg once or twice daily) to counteract this, although explanation will usually suffice.

Therapeutic response may be seen as early as 2–3 weeks, although a full response may not occur for at least 6–8 weeks. Increasing brain 5-HT appears to decrease panic, although, as described above, SSRIs and TCAs can exacerbate anxiety symptoms initially. This is an important concept to understand since simple explanation to the parent or child may help to increase their confidence and improve compliance. One theory for the initial exacerbation of anxiety and delayed panic-reducing effect suggests that it may be due to autoreceptor desensitization. When an SSRI is taken, it prevents 5-HT reuptake, leading to an increase in 5-HT at the synapse. This 5-HT also binds to the autoreceptors on the cell body, essentially turning off the firing of that neurone. The net effect is no change, or even a reduction in available 5-HT, and hence no therapeutic effect (or even a worsening) to start with. After 1–2 weeks these auto-receptors desensitize resulting in an increase in cell firing. The net effect of this is increased serotonergic throughput which is associated with the therapeutic effect (Chapter 3) *(Figure 15)*.

Benzodiazepines

Benzodiazepines are effective anxiolytics which are well tolerated and safe, but they do have a number of side-effects (*Table 28* and Chapter 3). Although they form an effective part of a treatment regime for panic disorder in adults, concern has been raised about prescribing benzodi-azepines for children because of the risk of dependency, tolerance, mis-use and their potential for causing behavioural disinhibition. Their role in juvenile panic disorder is very limited. It includes their short-term use (3–4 weeks) for cases of severe panic in which all other treatment approaches have failed and there is very considerable impairment and distress.

Separation anxiety disorder

Separation anxiety disorder is often seen as being synonymous with school refusal, although the latter is not a diagnosis in its own right but a description of associated behavioural problems. School refusal com-prises a heterogeneous group of anxiety and other child psychiatric dis-orders. Nevertheless, it is often one of the presenting features of separation anxiety disorder, and referral to a child psychiatrist tends to occur once school placement is at risk of breaking down. It is essential that a rapid response occurs in order to prevent secondary complica-tions within the family and for the child.

The features of separation anxiety disorder defined by DSM IV are in *Table 29.*

Table 28   Side-effects of benzodiazepines.

Fatigue
Drowsiness
Reduced concentration
Behavioural disinhibition
Psychomotor impairment
Impaired memory

Table 29   Features of separation anxiety disorder.

Developmentally inappropriate and excessive anxiety about separation from home or major attachment figures, as shown by excessive anxiety in at least 3 of the following situations:
    Separation or anticipation of separation
    Fear of loss of, or harm befalling, attachment figures
    Reluctance/refusal to go to school or elsewhere because of fear of separation
    Reluctance to be alone
    Reluctance/refusal to go to sleep alone or to sleep away from home
    Repeated nightmares about separation
    Repeated complaints of physical symptoms when separation occurs or is anticipated
Duration of at least 4 weeks
Causes significant distress or impairment of functioning

Prevalence

Separation anxiety disorder is relatively common and affects 2–4 per cent of the child and adolescent population. It is the most common anxiety disorder affecting pre-pubertal children.

Comorbidity

Comorbidity with other anxiety and mood disorders is common and frequently complicates the picture.

Aetiology

The aetiology of separation anxiety remains unclear but is likely to be multifactorial with genetic, biological, physiological and environmental factors all playing a role.

Assessment

A thorough assessment should include good collateral information from the school professionals involved, combined with a comprehensive evaluation of the child and family concerned. It is also useful to assess whether children have any somatic complaints and to compare their perceptions with their main carers as well as with those of health professionals who know the children.

Treatment

Psychological
Behavioural interventions, in particular graded exposure to the feared

situation (e.g. school attendance), are effective and can be used in combination with family intervention to ensure that avoidance behaviour is not being reinforced, or encouraged.

Psychopharmacological treatments
Earlier drug studies tended to use a wider diagnostic group that included anxious school-refusing children not necessarily fulfilling the current diagnostic criteria for separation anxiety disorder. One of the earlier trials looked at imipramine versus placebo and showed promising results,[88] but a later study failed to replicate these findings;[89] and a subsequent 12-week trial of low dose clomipramine (40–75 mg/day) did not show any therapeutic benefit. In a more recent open trial for the treatment of child and adolescent anxiety disorders including separation anxiety disorder fluoxetine showed clinical improvement. Further double-blind trials are clearly needed.

Of 21 children with a variety of anxiety disorders (overanxious disorder, social phobia or separation anxiety disorder) fluoxetine (mean dose 25.7 mg/day) was shown to produce a significant improvement.[90]

Generalized anxiety disorder

Children with generalized anxiety disorder (GAD) are persistent worriers. Their anxieties are not focused on any particular situation but tends to be about the future, the past, or their personal competence. The DSM IV diagnosis requires that the symptoms cause significant distress or impaired social functioning unlike ICD 10. Associated behaviours include self-consciousness, somatic symptoms (including headaches and abdominal pain), and difficulty relaxing (e.g. they startle easily and are tense).

The important features of GAD are shown in *Table 30*.

Prevalence

Approximately 3 per cent of children are affected with an increased incidence in adolescents. Higher socio-economic classes are over-

Table 30   Features of generalized anxiety disorder.

Excessive anxiety and worry about a number of events and activities
Worry difficult to control
Worry associated with restlessness, feeling on edge, being easily fatigued, having difficulty concentrating, irritability, muscle tension, sleep disturbance
Symptoms cause significant distress or impairment of functioning

represented and the sex ratio is approximately equal with a possible slightly increased preponderance in females.

Comorbidity

There is high comorbidity with other disorders, particularly separation anxiety disorder, mood disorders, and simple phobias.

Aetiology

The aetiology of GAD remains unclear although genetic and environmental factors are both implicated.

Neurochemical

There is some evidence from adult studies for noradrenergic, serotonergic and GABAergic dysfunction in GAD.

Of the noradrenergic receptors the α_2 is the one most clearly linked with anxiety. In adults with GAD there is a blunted growth hormone response to clonidine (a finding also reported in depression and panic disorder).[91] Other adult studies have also demonstrated decreased numbers of platelet α_2-adrenoreceptors. Both of these findings suggest subsensitivity of α_2-adrenoreceptors, perhaps reflecting downregulation of receptors secondary to excessive NA release. In children with anxiety disorders, however, the growth hormone response to clonidine challenge does not appear to be blunted, suggesting that there may be some differences from adults.[92]

Although 5-HT almost certainly has a role in anxiety and drugs which act on this system (SSRIs and the 5-HT$_{1A}$ agonist buspirone) are found to be effective as treatments, it is currently difficult to specify whether the problem in GAD is the result of a deficit or excess of this neurotransmitter. The levels of 5-HT in the cerebrospinal fluid of adult patients with GAD are reported to be lower than in normal controls. The 5-HT agonist m-CPP however causes increased anxiety responses in those with GAD suggesting hypersensitive receptors.[93]

GABA is the main inhibitory neurotransmitter in the brain. When GABA receptors are blocked, anxiety increases, and when they are stimulated, e.g. by benzodiazepines, it decreases. There is some evidence from adult studies that the sensitivity of GABA receptors is reduced in GAD.[94] SPECT studies similarly report a significant decrease in benzodiazepine receptor binding in patients with GAD compared with normal controls.[95]

Neuroanatomy

There have been very few imaging studies in adult patients with GAD and none in children. The adult studies suggest some involvement of several cortical regions and the basal ganglia.

In the 1980s, Gray proposed a neuroanatomical model for anxiety that seems to be particularly relevant for understanding many of the symptoms found in GAD. He called this the 'behavioural inhibition system'.[96] According to this model, the assessment of threat takes place in the septohippocampal area of the brain. The presence of threat activates the behavioural inhibition system, which results in increased arousal and the suppression of regular ongoing behaviours; a state very like GAD.

Assessment

Making the diagnosis of GAD in children and adolescents requires completing a very careful assessment of the young person, the family and the school environment to ascertain the nature of the worry and how this affects their everyday functioning.

Treatment

Psychological

Evaluative research of psychological treatments appears to be limited to one large study that used modified CBT over a 16-week period in children with mixed anxiety disorders, although the most prevalent primary diagnosis was GAD. Results showed promising therapeutic benefit compared to a waiting list group, an effect which was maintained at 1-year of follow-up.

Psychopharmacological treatment

Once again the changing nosology for child anxiety disorders has meant that little research has been conducted on this relatively new diagnosis. Previous studies used the diagnosis of overanxious disorder and have not produced promising results. One study compared alprazolam with placebo and showed no benefit.[97] In an open study of fluoxetine on 21 children and adolescents with a range of anxiety disorders described earlier[90] improvements were found but clearly more specific controlled trials are warranted.

There is also some suggestion that buspirone may be effective in the treatment of child and adolescent GAD. In adults it has significant benefits over benzodiazepines in that it has a limited side-effect profile, no potential for abuse, and no known withdrawal reaction. It does however take longer for its anxiolytic effects to emerge, e.g. 2–3 weeks (*Table 31*

Table 31   Advantages of buspirone.

No withdrawal reaction
No memory or psychomotor impairment
No potential for abuse
Side-effects relatively benign, e.g. dizziness, fatigue and GI upset

and Chapter 2). This needs to be emphasized in order to ensure compliance. Buspirone may also require twice-daily dosing due to its short half-life which ranges from 2–10 h.

Post-traumatic stress disorder

Although post-traumatic stress disorder (PTSD) is a well-established diagnosis among the adult population it was first applied to children and adolescents with the revision of DSM to DSM III R in1987. *Table 32* summarizes the four criteria which must be met to establish a DSM IV diagnosis of PTSD.

The diagnosis can be applied to children under the age of 5 years. The exposure trauma should constitute actual death, serious injury or threat to the child's physical integrity, or to that of loved ones. Overwhelming events should take the form of either a single, unexpected event or a long-standing and repetitive series of events such as severe physical, emotional, or sexual abuse. It has been argued that the event itself does not need to be directly experienced by the child but can take the form of an indirect trauma such as witnessing violent acts.

Children often present with symptoms of lethargy and disinterest that reflect a general numbing of responsiveness. It is important that this is understood by the carers and professionals concerned and not misinterpreted. They may also withdraw socially or exhibit symptoms of hyperarousal which may be manifested as impaired concentration, sleep disturbance, and irritability.[98]

Prevalence

It is hard to find precise prevalence figures for PTSD in children. It is being increasingly recognized that a significant number of children do witness serious domestic violence which may lead to the symptoms of PTSD. For physically abused children, rates of PTSD using DSM criteria

Table 32   Required criteria for DSM IV diagnosis of PTSD.

Exposure to life-threatening event
Subsequent re-experiencing of event (intrusive thoughts or memories, dreams or, less commonly, flashbacks)
Consequent avoidance of traumatic reminders or numbing of general responsiveness
Persistent increased arousal, e.g. sleep disturbances, irritability, difficulty concentrating, hypervigilance, exaggerated startle responses and outbursts of aggression

may reach prevalence rates of 20 per cent; and for sexually abused children, 44 per cent.

Comorbidity

Comorbidity with other mood or anxiety disorders or substance misuse is a frequent finding.

Aetiology

Several neurotransmitter systems appear to be important in this condition, including NA, 5-HT and the endogenous opioid system, although again most of the evidence comes from adult studies.[99] Recently, there have been some intriguing results suggesting that adults who were sexually abused as children have reduced hippocampal volume compared with matched controls, possibly secondary to increased levels of cortisol.[100] Although only preliminary these findings do fit with other data suggesting similar abnormalities in war veterans with PTSD and emphasize that trauma through early abuse may have major long-term implications.

Assessment

A family assessment initially followed by individual assessment and collaborating histories from significant others allows the clinician to establish not only a therapeutic relationship but also to demarcate the significant events leading to the disorder.

Treatment

Although the occurrence of PTSD in children and adolescents is increasingly well documented there are very few treatment studies in this population.

Psychological
Psychological treatment, in particular CBT, is generally considered to be the mainstay of treatment for this disorder in children,[101] although there is little evaluation of its efficacy.

Eye movement desensitization (EMDR) is a relatively new technique proposed as a treatment for PTSD in adults. Results have been promising although its theoretical basis seems less clear. The technique requires the person to recall traumatic memories while following a series of tracking eye movements. They are first asked to rehearse negative associated thoughts and to monitor subsequent emotional and physical experiences stimulated through the process until they experience a reduction in distress measured using a subjective units of disturbance scale (SUDS). They are then asked to rehearse a positive belief during eye movement tracking in order to 'install' the belief. One hypothesis suggests that EMDR facilitates an accelerated process of learning assuming that the original information fails to be incorporated adaptively at the time of trauma due to the overwhelming nature of the experience. Others propose that it 'overwrites' the memories causing PTSD.[102] Although the results of EMDR are of interest its use in children or adolescents with PTSD has yet to be evaluated.

Psychopharmacological treatment

The only drug currently licensed for the treatment of adults with PTSD is sertraline (in the USA) and the disorder is at an even earlier stage of evaluation for children. Management is, therefore, at the discretion of the clinician and should be considered if there are significant symptoms of anxiety and/or depression. SSRIs seem to be particularly effective at reducing the symptoms of numbness experienced in PTSD, unlike other drugs that have been studied.[103] Contrary to initial assumptions therapeutic effects can be seen within 2 weeks of treatment. Undesirable side-effects of arousal and insomnia, which are particularly intolerable for PTSD patients, can be treated with trazadone (which reverses the insomnia) or similar sedating drugs.

There has been some interest in the use of adrenergic drugs in PTSD. Open trials of clonidine (an α_2 adrenergic agonist) showed a reduction in traumatic nightmares, hypervigilance, insomnia, and angry outbursts, along with an improvement of mood and concentration.[104] These suggest that α_2 agonists may be particulary helpful in treating the symptoms of hyperarousal in children with PTSD.

Specific phobia

Specific phobias are common in adulthood and phobias include for example the fear of needles, animals, and public speaking. They can be categorized into the types listed in *Table 33*.

Prevalence

Specific phobias affect between 2 per cent and 4 per cent of children and in adolescents with an equal sex ratio.

Table 33   Specific phobia types.

Animal
Natural/environmental
Situational
Blood-injection injury
Mixed

Specific phobias have an early onset (5 years) and have low rates of comorbidity compared with other anxiety disorders. Their aetiology can involve phobia-specific traumatic events, learnt behaviour from parents or peers and a genetic predisposition.

Assessment

When considering a diagnosis of specific phobia it is important to distinguish the symptoms from normal specific fears which are very common throughout childhood. Both DSM IV and ICD 10 require that the feared object must be either avoided or endured with intense anxiety which emphasizes the point that they have a significant impact on the child's life.

Treatment

Psychological
Graded exposure provides the mainstay of treatment for specific phobia, although this is often used in combination with other cognitive-behavioural techniques.

Psychopharmacological treatment
There is no evidence for the efficacy of drugs in the treatment of specific phobias although it has been shown that benzodiazepines may help adults engage in exposure therapy by reducing anticipatory anxiety. Very recently paroxetine has been shown to reduce anxiety measures in adults with specific phobias and so could be considered as an adjunctive treatment for children with disabling specific phobias.

References

1 Bjerkenstedt L, Flyckt L, Overo KF, Lingiaerde O. Relationship between clinical effects, serum drug concentration and serotonin uptake inhibition in depressed patients treated with citalopram. *Eur J Clin Pharmacol* (1985) **28:** 553–7.

2 Shiloh R, Nutt DJ, Weizman A. *Atlas of psychiatric pharmacotherapy*. London: Martin Dunitz Publishers, 1999.

3 American Psychiatric Association. *Diagnostic and statistical manual of mental disorders*, 4th edn. Washington DC: American Psychiatric Association, (1994) 317–66.

4 World Health Organization. *The ICD–10 classification of mental and behavioural disorders: clinical descriptions and diagnostic guidelines*. Geneva: World Health Organization, 1992: 110–31.

5 Rutter M, Taylor E, Hersor L. *Child and adolescent psychiatry modern approaches*. Oxford: Blackwell Science, 1993.

6 Strober M. Mixed mania associated with tricyclic antidepressant therapy in prepubertal delusional depression: three cases. *J Child Adolesc Psychopharmacol* (1998) **8**(3): 181–5.

7 Anderson JC, Williams S, McGee R, Silva PA. DSM-III disorders in preadolescent children: prevalence in a large sample from the general population. *Arch Gen Psychiatry* (1987) **44:** 69–76.

8 Fleming J, Offord DR. Epidemiology of childhood depressive disorders: a critical review. *J Am Acad Child Adolesc Psychiatry* (1990) **29:** 571–80.

9 Velez CN, Johnson J, Cohen P. A longtitudinal analysis of selected risk factors for childhood psychopathology. *J Am Acad Child Adolesc Psychiatry* (1989) **28:** 861–4.

10 Cooper PJ, Goodyer I. A community study of depression in adolescent girls. I: Estimates of symptom and syndrome prevalence (1993) *Br J Psychiatry* **163:** 369–74.

11 McClure GMG. Suicide in children and adolescents in England and Wales 1960–1990. *Br J Psychiatry* (1994) **165:** 510–14.

12 Office of Population Census and Surveys 1990 mortality statistics, cause: England and Wales. 1990 Series DH2, 17. HMSO, London.

13 Brent D, Perper JA, Goldstein C, et al. Risk factors for adolescent suicide: a comparison of adolescent suicide victims and suicide inpatients *Arch Gen Psychiatry* (1988) **45:** 581–8.

14 Schildkraut JJ. The catecholamine theory of affective disorders: a review of the evidence. *Am J Psychiatry* (1965) **122:** 509–22.

15 Delgado PL, Charney DS, Price LH, et al. Serotonin function and the mechanism of antidepressant action: reversal of antidepressant induced remission by rapid depletion of plasma tryptophan. *Arch Gen Psychiatry* (1990) **47:** 411–19.

16 Kowatch RA, Devous MD, Harvey DC, et al. A spect HMPAO. A study of regional cerebral blood flow in depressed adolescents and normal controls. *Prog Neuropsychopharmacol Biol Psychiatry* (1999) **3:** 643–56.

17 Steingard RJ, Renshaw PF, Yurgelun-Todd, et al. Structural abnormalities in brain magnetic resonance images of depressed children. *J Am Acad Child Adolesc Psychiatry* (1996) **35:** 307–11.

18 Harrington RC, Fudge H, Rutter M, et al. Child and adult depression: a test of continuities with data from a family study. *Br J Psychiatry* (1993) **162:** 627–33.

19 Goodyer IM, Cooper P, Vize C, Ashby L. Depression in 11–16 year-old girls: the role of past parental psychopathology and exposure to recent life events. *J Child Psychol Psychiatry* (1993) **34**(7): 1103–15.

20 Seligman MEP. *Helplessness: on depression, development and death.* San Francisco, CA: Freeman, 1975.

21 Beck AT, Rush AJ, Shaw BF, Emery G. *Cognitive therapy of depression.* New York: Guildford Press, 1979.

22 Rutter M, Quinton D. Parental psychiatric disorder: effects on children. *Psychol Med* (1984) **14**(4): 853–80.

23 Daly JM, Wilens T. The use of tricyclic antidepressants in children and adolescents. *Pediatr Clin North Am* (1998) **45**(5): 1123–35.

24 Birmaher B. Childhood and adolescent depression: a review of the past 10 years. Part II. *J Am Acad Child Adolesc Psychiatry* (1996) **35**(12): 1575–83.

25 Birmaher B. Should we use antidepressant medications for children and adolescents with depressive disorders? *Psychopharmacol Bull* (1998) **34**(1): 35–9.

26 Geller B, Reising D, Leonard HL, et al. Critical review of tricyclic antidepressant use in children and adolescents. *J Am Acad Child Adolesc Psychiatry* (1999) **38**(5): 513–16.

27 Varley CK, McClellan J. Case study: two additional sudden deaths with tricyclic antidepressants. *J Am Acad Child Adolesc Psychiatry* (1997) **36**(3): 390–4.

28 Kutcher, SP. Affective disorders in children and adolescents: a critical clinically relevant review. In Walsh BT, ed. *Child psychopharmacology.* Washington, DC (1998); 91–114.

29 Ryan ND, Varma D. Child and adolescent mood disorders – experience with serotonin-based therapies. *Biol Psychiatry* (1998) **44**(5): 336–40.

30 Emslie GJ, Rush AJ, Weinberg WA. A double-blind, randomized, placebo-controlled trial of fluoxetine in children and adolescents with depression. *Arch Gen Psychiatry* (1997) **54**(11): 1031–7.

31 Simeon J, DiNicola V, Ferguson H, et al. Adolescent depression: a placebo-controlled fluoxetine treatment study and follow up. *Prog Neuropsychopharm Biol Psychiatry* (1990) **14:** 791–5.

32 Kowatch RA, Carmody TJ, Emslie GJ, et al. Prediction of response to fluoxetine and placebo in children and adolescents with major depression: a hypothesis generating study. *J Affect Disord* (1999) **54**(3): 269–76.

33 Bostic JQ, Wilens TE, Spencer T, et al. Antidepressant treatment of juvenile depression. *Int J Psychiatry Clin Pract* (1999) **3:** 171–9.

34 Wagner KD, Birmaher B, Carlson G, et al. *Safety of paroxetine and imipramine in the treatment of adolescent depression.* 151st Meeting of the American Psychiatric Association, Toronto, May, 1998. APA, Washington DC.

35 Rodríguez Ramos P, Díos Vega J, San Sebastian Cabases J, et al. Effects of paroxetine in depressed adolescents. *Eur J Clin Res* (1996) **8:** 49–61.

36 Rey Sanchez F, Gutierrez Casares JR. Paroxetine in children with major depressive disorder: an open trial. *J Am Acad Child Adolesc Psychiatry.* (1997) **36**(10): 1443–7.

37 McConville BJ, Minnery KL, Sorter MT, et al. An open study of the effects of sertraline on adolescent major depression. *J Child Adolesc Psychopharmacol* (1996) **6**(1): 41–51.

38 Tierney E, Joshi PT, Llinas JF, et al. Sertraline for major depression in children and adolescents: preliminary clinical subtypes. *J Child Adolesc Psychopharmacol* (1995) **5:** 13–27.

39 Ambrosini PJ, Wagner KD, Biederman J, et al. Multicenter open-label sertraline study in adolescent outpatients with major depression. *J Am Acad Child Adolesc Psychiatry* (1999) **38**(5): 566–72.

40 Apter JT, Ratzoni G, King RA, et al. Fluvoxamine open-label treatment of adolescent inpatients with obsessive-compulsive disorder or depression. *J Am Acad Child Adolesc Psychiatry* (1994) **33:** 342–8.

41 Cosgrove PVF. Fluvoxamine in the treatment of depressive illness in children and adolescents. *J Psychopharmacol* (1994) **8**(2): 118–23.

42 Guile JM. Sertraline-induced behavioural activation during the treatment of an adolescent with major depression. *J Child Adolesc Psychopharmacol* (1996) **6**(4): 281–5.

43 Go FS, Malley EE, Birmaher B, Rosenberg DR. Manic behaviours associated with fluoxetine in three 12- to 18-year olds with obsessive-compulsive disorder. *J Child Adolesc Psychopharmacol* (1998) **8**(1): 73–80.

44 King RA, Riddle MA, Chappell PB, et al. Emergence of self-destructive phenomena in children and adolescents during fluoxetine treatment. *J Am Acad Child Adolesc Psychiatry* (1991) **30:** 179–86.

45 Goodnick PJ, Jorge CM, Hunter TA, et al. *Nefazodone in adolescent depression.* Proceedings of the American Psychiatric Association. Toronto, June 1998: 253, APA, Washington, DC.

46 Mandoki MW, Tapia MR, Sumner GS, Parker JL. Venlafaxine in the treatment of children and adolescents with major depression. *Psychopharmacol Bull* (1997) **33**(1): 149–54.

47 Anderson JM, Nutt DJ, Deakin JFW, on behalf of the Consensus Meeting and endorsed by British Association for Psychopharmacology. Evidence-based guidelines for treating depressive disorders with antidepressants: a revision of 1993 British Association for Psychopharmacology guidelines. *J Psychopharmacol* (2000) **14:** 113–20.

48 Nemeroff CB. Augmentation regimens for depression. *J Clin Psychiatry* (1991) **52**(suppl): 21–7.

49 Panay N, Studd JW. The psychotherapeutic effects of oestro-

gens. *Gynaecol Endocrinol* (1998) **12**(5): 353–65.

50 Walter G, Rey JM, Mitchell PB. Practitioner review: electroconvulsive therapy in adolescents. *J Child Psychol Psychiatry Allied Disciplines* (1999) **40**(3): 325–34.

51 Glue P, Costello MJ, Pert A, et al. Regional neurotransmitter responses after acute and chronic electroconvulsive shock. *Psychopharmacology* (1989) **100**: 60–5.

52 Traversa G, Spila-Alegiani S, Arpino C, Ferrara M. Prescription of neuroleptics for children and adolescents in Italy. *J Child Adolesc Psychopharmacol* (1998) **8**(3): 175–80.

53 Kumra S, Herion D, Jacobsen LK, et al. Case study: risperidone induced hepatotoxicity in paediatric patients. *J Am Acad Child Adolesc Psychiatry* (1997) **36**(5): 701–5.

54 Hollander E, Kwon JH, Stein DJ, et al. Obsessive-compulsive and spectrum disorders: overview and quality of life issues. *J Clin Psychiatry* (1996) **57:** 3–6.

55 Flament MF, Koby F, Rapoport JL, et al. Childhood obsessive-compulsive disorder: a prospective follow up study. *J Child Psychol Psychiatry* (1990) **31:** 363–80.

56 Leonard HL, Swedo SE, Rapoport JL, et al. Treatment of obsessive-compulsive disorder with clomipramine and desipramine in children and adolescents. *Arch Gen Psychiatry* (1989) **46:** 1088–92.

57 Swedo SE, Rapoport JL, Leonard H, et al. Obsessive-compulsive disorder in children and adolescents. Clinical phenomenology of 70 consecutive cases. *Arch Gen Psychiatry* (1989) **46:** 335–40.

58 Flament MF, Rapoport JL, Berg CJ, et al. Clomipramine treatment of childhood obsessive-compulsive disorder. A double-blind controlled study. *Arch Gen Psychiatry* (1985) **42:** 977–83.

59 Sallee FR, Richman H, Beach K, et al. Platelet serotonin transporter in children and adolescents with obsessive-compulsive disorder or Tourette's syndrome. *J Am Acad Child Adolesc Psychiatry* (1996) **35:** 1647–56.

60 Swedo SE, Rapoport JL, Cheslow DL, et al. High prevalence of obsessive-compulsive symptoms in patients with Sydenham's chorea. *Am J Psychiatry* (1989) **146:** 246–9.

61 Swedo SE, Leonard H, Shapiro MB, et al. Sydenham's chorea: physical and psychological symptoms of Saint Vitus's dance. *Paediatrics* (1993) **91:** 706–13.

62 Perlmutter SJ, Leitman SF, Garvey MA, et al. Therapeutic plasma exchange and intravenous immunoglobulin for obsessive-compulsive disorder and tic disorders in childhood. *Lancet* (1999) **354:** 1153–8.

63 Peterson B, Leckman J, Tucker D, et al. Preliminary findings of anti-streptoccocal titres and basal ganglia volumes in tic, obsessive-compulsive and attention deficit/hyperactivity disorders. *Arch Gen Psychiatry* (2000) **57:** 364–72.

64 Baxter LR, Jeffrey M, Schwartz MD, et al. Caudate glucose metabolic rate changes with both drug and behaviour therapy for obsessive-compulsive disorder. *Arch Gen Psychiatry* (1992) **46:** 681–9.

65 Gilbert AR, Moore GJ, Keshaven MS, et al. Decrease in thalamic volumes of paediatric patients with OCD who are taking paroxetine. *Arch Gen Psychiatry* (2000) **57:** 449–56.

66 Rosenberg DR, Benazon NR, Gilbert A, et al. Thalamic volume in paediatric OCD patients before and after cognitive behavioural

therapy. *Biol Psychiatry* (2000) **48:** 294–300.

67 Giedd JN, Rapaport JL, Garvey MA, et al. MRI assessment of children with obsessive compulsive disorder or tics associated with streptococcal injection. *Am J Psychiatry* (2000) **157:** 281–3.

68 Riddle M. Obsessive-compulsive disorder in children and adolescents. *Br J Psychiatry Suppl* (1998) **35:** 91–6.

69 De Vaughn-Geiss J, Moroz G, Biederman J, et al. Clomipramine hydrochoride in childhood and adolescent obsessive-compulsive disorder: a multi-center trial. *J Am Acad Child Adolesc Psychiatry* (1992) **31:** 45–9.

70 Riddle MA, Scahill L, King RA, et al. Double-blind, crossover trial of fluoxetine and placebo in children and adolescents with obsessive-compulsive disorder. *J Am Acad Child Adolesc Psychiatry* (1992) **31:** 1062–9.

71 March JS, Biederman J, Wolkow R, et al. Sertraline in children and adolescents with obsessive-compulsive disorder: a multi-center randomized controlled trial. *JAMA* (1998) **280:** 1752–6.

72 Thomsen PU. Child and adolescent obsessive-compulsive disorder treated with citalopram: findings from an open trial of 23 cases. *J Child Adolesc Psychopharmacol* (1997) **7:** 157–66.

73 Dryden-Edwards RC, Reiss AL. Differential response of psychotic and obsessive symptoms to risperidone in an adolescent. *J Child Adolesc Psychopharmacol* (1996) **6:** 139–45.

74 Magee WJ, Eaton WW, Wittchen H, et al. Agoraphobia, simple phobia, and social phobia in the national comorbidity survey. *Arch Gen Psychiatry* (1996) **59:** 159–68.

75 Bell CJ, Malizia AL, Nutt DJ. The neurobiology of social phobia. *Eur Arch Psychiatry Clin Neurosci* (1999) **249:** S11–S18.

76 Nutt DJ, Bell CJ, Malizia AL. Brain mechanisms of social anxiety disorder. *J Clin Psychiatry* (1998) **59** (17): 4–9.

77 Hollander E, Kwon J, Weiller F, et al. Serotonergic function in social phobia: comparison to normal control and obsessive-compulsive disorder subjects. *Psychiatry Res* (1998) **79:** 213–17.

78 Tiihonen J, Kuikka J, Bergstrom K, et al. Dopamine reuptake site densities in patients with social phobia. *Am J Psychiatry* (1997) **154:** 239–42.

79 Black B, Udhe TW. Psychiatric characteristics of children with selective mutism: a pilot study. *J Am Acad Child Adolesc Psychiatry* (1995) **34:** 847–56.

80 Birmaher D, Waterman GS, Ryan N, et al. Fluoxetine for childhood anxiety disorders. *J Am Acad Child Adolesc Psychiatry* (1994) **33:** 993–9.

81 Dummit ES, Klein RG, Tancer NK, et al. Fluoxetine treatment of children with selective mutism: an open trial. *J Am Acad Child Adolesc Psychiatry* (1996) **35:** 615–21.

82 Pitts FM, McClure JN. Lactate metabolism in anxiety neurosis. *N Engl J Med* (1967) **277:** 1329–36.

83 Bell C, Nutt D. Serotonin and panic. *Br J Psych* (1998) 172; 4650171.

84 Nutt DJ, Glue P, Lawson C, Wilson S. Flumazenil provocation of panic attacks. *Arch Gen Psychiatry* (1990) **47:** 917–25.

85 Malizia A, Cunningham VJ, Bell CJ, et al. Decreased brain GABA-A benzodiazepine receptor binding in panic disorder. *Arch Gen Psychiatry* (1998) **55:** 715–20.

86 Bradley SJ, Hood J. Psychiatri-

cally referred adolescents with panic attacks: presenting symptoms, stressors and comorbidity. *J Am Acad Child Adolesc Psychiatry* (1993) **32:** 826–9.

87 Ollendick TH. Panic disorder in children and adolescents. *J Clin Child Psychol* (1998) **27:** 234–45.

88 Gittelman-Klein R, Klein DF. Controlled imipramine treatment of school phobia. *Arch Gen Psychiatry* (1971) **25:** 204–7.

89 Klein RG, Kopiewicz HS, Kanner A. Imipramine treatment of children with separation anxiety disorder. *J Am Acad Child Adolesc Psychiatry* (1992) **31:** 21–8.

90 Birmaher B, Waterman GS, Ryan N, et al. Fluoxetine for childhood anxiety disorders. *J Am Acad Child Adolesc Psychiatry* (1994) **33:** 993–9.

91 Abelson JL, Glitz D, Cameron OG, et al. Blunted growth hormone response to clonidine in patients with generalised anxiety disorder. *Arch Gen Psychiatry* (1990) **48:** 157–62.

92 Sallee FR, Richman H, Sethuramen G, et al. Clonidine challenge in childhood anxiety disorder. *J Am Acad Child Adolesc Psychiatry* (1998) **37:** 655–62.

93 Germine M, Goddard AW, Woods SW, et al. Anger and anxiety responses to m-CPP in generalised anxiety disorder. *Biol Psychiatry* (1992) **32:** 457–61.

94 Cowley DS, Roy-Byrne PP, Hommer DW, et al. Benzodiazepine sensitivity in anxiety disorders. *Biol Psych* (1991) **29:** 57A.

95 Tiihonen J, Kuikka J, Rasansen P, et al. Cerebral benzodiazepine receptor binding and distribution in generalised anxiety disorder: a fractal analysis. *Mol Psychiatry* (1997) **2:** 463–71.

96 Gray JA. The neuropsychological basis of anxiety. In Last CG, Hersen M, eds. *Handbook of anxiety disorders.* New York: Pergamon Press, 1988: 10–37.

97 Simeon JG, Ferguson HB, Knott V, et al. Clinical, cognitive and neurophysiological effects of alprazolam in children and adolescents with overanxious and avoidant disorders. *J Am Acad Child Adolesc Psychiatry* (1992) **31:** 29–33.

98 Stallard P, Law F. Screening and psychological debriefing of adolescent survivors of life-threatening events. *Br J Psychiatry* (1993) **163:** 660–5.

99 Nutt DJ, Ballenger J, McFarlane A, et al. The psychobiology of posttraumatic stress disorder. *J Clin Psychiatry* (2000) **61:** 24–9, 30–2.

100 Bremner JD, Randall P, Vermetten E, et al. Magnetic resonance imaging-based measurement of hippocampal volume in posttraumatic stress disorder related to childhood physical and sexual abuse—a preliminary report. *Biol Psychiatry* (1997) **41:** 23–32.

101 Cohen J, March J, Berliner L. Treatment guidelines for PTSD in children and adolescents. In Foa E, ed. ISTSS *treatment guidelines for PTSD.* Chicago: ISTSS, in press.

102 Shapiro F. Accelerated information processing. The model as a working hypothesis. In: *Eye movement desensitisation and reprocessing: basic principles, protocols and procedures.* New York: Guildford Press, 1995.

103 Donelly CL, Arnaya-Jackson L, March JS. Psychoparmacology and paediatric post-traumatic stress disorder. *J Child Adolesc Psychopharmacol* (1990) **9:** 203–20.

104 Friedman MJ. Current and future drug treatment for posttraumatic stress disorder patients. *Psychiatric Ann* (1998) **28:** 461–8.

Index